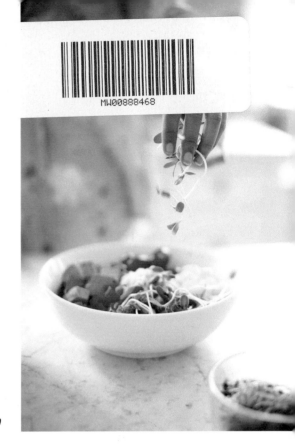

counting colors,
NOT CALORIES

A SHIFT FROM RESTRICTION AND SCARCITY TO ABUNDANCE AND BEAUTY

By Sara McGlothlin

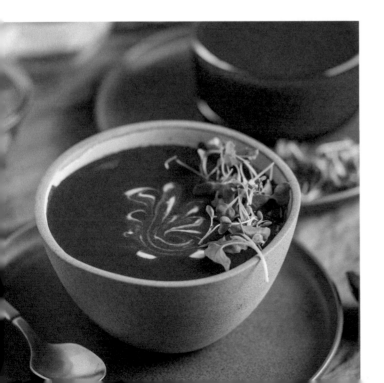

D E D I C A T I O N :

For Mason, who makes my life more colorful than I could have imagined.

Counting Colors, Not Calories

A Shift from Restriction and Scarcity to Abundance and Beauty

©2022, All rights reserved.

ISBN: 979-8-338-44556-3

By Sara McGlothlin

sara@healthified.com

For permission requests, please email the author.

Cover image by Ash Carr

Author headshot by Haley Tibbs

Food photography by Sara McGlothlin

Book design by Shay Design

An important note to the reader: This book is intended to provide helpful information on the topics discussed. This book should not be used to treat or diagnose a health issue or condition. Please seek advice from your physician or other medical professional before implementing any health program or treatment.

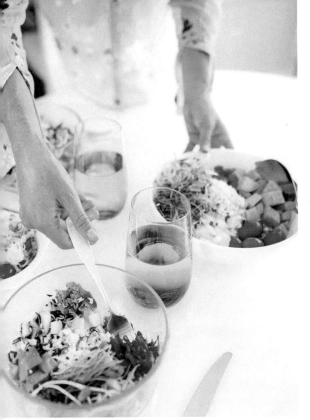

TABLE OF
contents

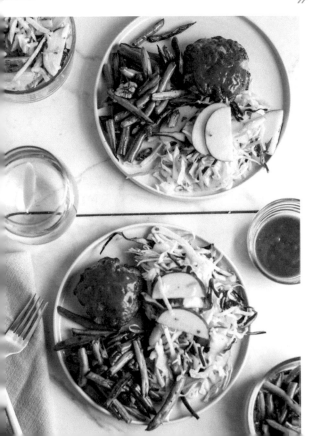

preface

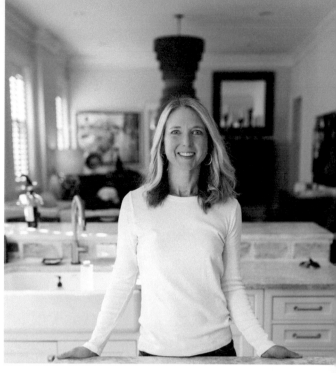

I was biking the streets of Amsterdam when the concept of my Counting Colors philosophy—which started out as a purely nutritional mantra—evolved into something more abstract. *Look at all the colors*, I remember thinking to myself as I noticed everything from the flowers to the facades of people's homes. During this three-month backpacking excursion with my husband, I had never felt so present, and although traveling to this degree comes with its own stressors, what I did not carry with me was the everyday stress from life back home. I returned feeling lighter (both physically and mentally) and more aligned. Not only did the stubborn pounds I had worked to lose for fifteen years through a strict diet and exercise regimen seem to melt off me, but I was also *happy* and more mindful of my surroundings. Happiness had mostly been an emotion I had known in response to something, especially (I hate to admit) when I felt in control of my physical body. What I have come to learn in the years since is that you do not need to travel overseas to experience similar changes in mindset. That is the beautiful thing about practicing presence—you can do it anywhere at any time.

After the trip, I worked tirelessly over the subsequent months to get it all out of my head and onto *something*. I decided to launch Counting Colors as an online course, and it began to take shape in webinars and workbook material. And because I am a nutrition coach after all, over fifty recipes followed suit. I was nervous to share this idea with others, and a little scared it might be perceived as too "woo-woo" in a world where people want instant gratification and a quick fix, especially when it comes to what to eat, how to exercise, and other forms of self-care that will lead to personal betterment. I know this because I used to be one of those people.

However, after a couple successful rounds of hosting the program, I knew it was time to bring it to a larger audience. In the pages that follow, I share an inspirational idea I am extremely passionate about. In terms of how to take care of yourself, I want to shout from the rooftops, "Stop looking outside of yourself, go inward instead! You already have everything you need.

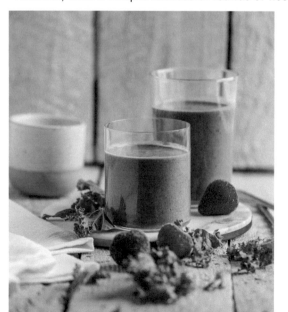

The digital version of the Counting Colors course is still available today on my website, but I have composed all of the information and some of the reflection exercises amongst these pages. Please visit ***www.countingcolors.com*** to learn more.

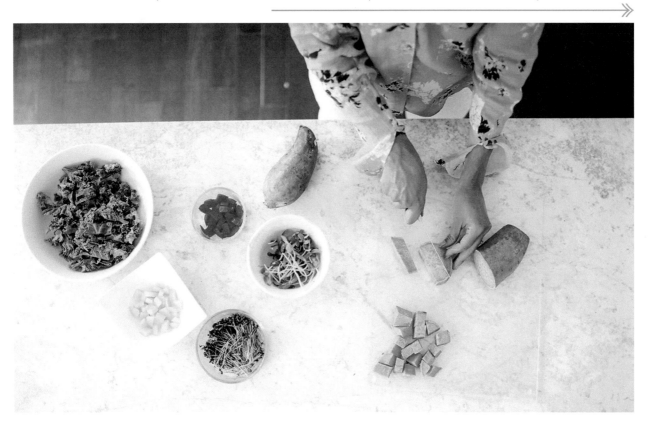

introduction

We all have a relationship with food. Not only is food a large part of culture and tradition from a societal perspective, but individually, it can be a relationship that roots us back to childhood. As the years go by, it can then become more deeply entangled with who we are and how we live. Given that biology prescribes we eat multiple times per day, it is something that inevitably shows up in our daily lives. Some people exemplify a more objective relationship with food (i.e. food as fuel), while others possess a more emotional attachment to it. And sometimes—as I have seen in myself and in others—our behavior around food can mirror (often subconsciously) certain deep-seated beliefs we hold about ourselves. As Geneen Roth states in her book *Women, Food, and God*, "How you eat is how you live."[1]

While I hope this book inspires you to embrace a more positive path to better health and happiness, I have to be honest: I also wrote *Counting Colors* for me. Not only was the creative process extremely cathartic, but through the writing and reading and editing, I learned something—and the insights kept coming. It is like Brené Brown explained in the introduction of her latest book *Dare to Lead*: "Write the book you need to read."[2] Because it is true what they say: Health is a journey, not a destination. I am a work in progress, practicing this philosophy every day.

This has been my journey; my evolution from fear to love. I share my story knowing that there are others who have similar struggles, and if my story can help one person, then my heart will be happy. I think that is the beautiful thing about the human condition: If we have the courage to convey our vulnerabilities, share our challenges, while connecting with others, our stories might just help someone else.

I initially adopted "count colors, not calories" as a nutritional mantra, especially when working with my health coaching clients who had a history of dieting, crunching numbers, and restricting themselves to a standardized way of eating based on a math equation. "Counting colors" epitomizes the shift of releasing the rules and eating more real, whole foods—the foods found in nature, containing various nutrients, which are represented by different colors. When you replace those brown and white processed foods that largely characterize the Standard American Diet with the natural foods our bodies were built to consume, you start to notice a beautiful collage of colors on your plate. Your plate becomes a canvas on which to create, which in turn influences a more mindful approach to eating.

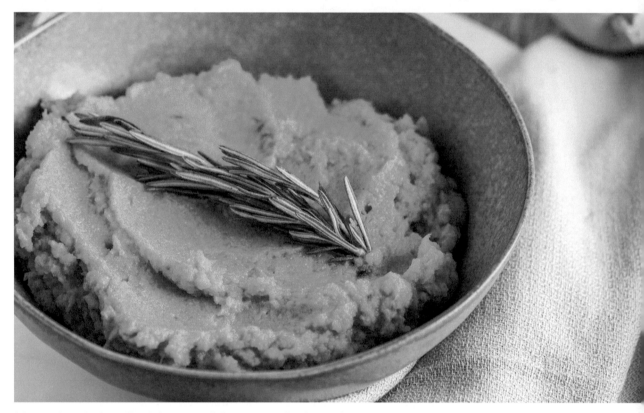

I have already described the exact "aha moment" when this catchphrase of encouragement in the realm of nutrition expanded to the possibility that it could pertain to various aspects of holistic health. In other words, it not only describes the shifts I would love for you to adopt in terms of what you are eating but also in how you are eating: to view food more beautifully and improve the relationship you have with it.

This shift basically became one big analogy for life and suddenly turned into more of a philosophy than a mantra. The philosophy not only embodies my personal journey with food but also better explains my evolution toward more mindfulness (both on the plate and off) and strengthening my intuition while simultaneously softening my ego.

While I will get into it more in later chapters, we all have an ego and an intuition. Your ego is essentially your thoughts; what I like to call that noisy mental chatter that often feels like a broken record in the background of your mind as you navigate throughout the day. Your ego is quite the elaborate storyteller. Its tendency is to cause unnecessary stress and anxiety, attaching to situations and circumstances that either are not happening in the present moment or will never happen in the future. In other words, it lies to you all day long. Ironically, your ego's job is to keep you safe, but in actuality, it keeps you scared. Without consciousness and awareness for your ego, it continues to shape a lens framed by fear. Interestingly enough, your ego is not "you," but it does tend to play a large role in creating your image of "self." We are so intertwined with this voice in our heads, however, that for much of our lives, it can *feel* like that is who we are—but this is not the case.

Your intuition is your inner being, the pure essence of who you are. We all have that peaceful, calm, all-knowing part of ourselves, but it simply gets overshadowed by the fearful ego over the years. A major aspect of the Counting Colors philosophy encourages you to tap into and strengthen your intuition, while releasing your ego. While it is not possible to completely get rid of your ego, it is possible to mute its influence over your mindset. One of the main ways we do this is through awareness.

For the sake of my analogy, your intuition (the calm, peaceful, mindful) is represented by color, while your ego (the fear, scarcity, lack) is embodied by black and white. When I think of this parallel, I am reminded of an analogy pertaining to mindfulness and meditation: that no matter how dark and stormy your thoughts, there is always blue sky beyond the clouds. According to spiritual teacher and Buddhist Pema Chodron, "You are the sky, everything else is just the weather."

To take the analogy a step further, when I think of color, I think of light. By definition, color is the element that is produced when light, striking an object, is reflected back to the eye. This is a major component of the Counting Colors message: to shed light on what is real and reveal what is true. I do not want to tell you what is true for you, per se, but rather help guide you to discover what is true for yourself. In other words, to instigate that shift in your perception and encourage you to embrace your authenticity. A process that starts with your relationship with food, and unfolds to include the relationship you have with yourself, eventually evolving to a higher state of consciousness. The text *A Course in Miracles* states that "miracles are seen in light."[3] This will take some inner work, but it will be worth it.

Before we dive into everything, there are a couple over-arching themes I will be addressing:

SHIFTING FROM FEAR TO LOVE

THE ART OF NON-JUDGMENT

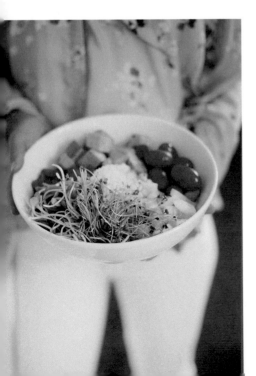

Judgement is when we attach labels to thoughts, objects, ideas, concepts, and occurrences, which in turn moralizes them into categories of "good" versus "bad." As human beings, we judge constantly, whether it is with our behavior and choices or other people's behavior and choices, and as women, we especially place judgement on food. It is important to realize that much of the time, what we are judging is not inherently good or bad at all; this is simply how we are perceiving it. How we perceive everything—not just our physical health—is so largely tied to our core values, beliefs, and "stories." I will elaborate on this idea of "your story" after sharing my own (and have you reflect on yours as well). Our respective health journeys have their own sets of stories and beliefs; therefore, when we take a step back to become more of an objective observer, it can help "shed light" on what is true. I hope you can see how all of this is coming together!

The Counting Colors philosophy encompasses a few different facets, which characterize an evolution in your holistic health:

The physical. The nutritional information rooted in science. If I was to over-simplify my food philosophy, it would be to eat real food. Eating whole, real, *colorful* foods, while balancing your blood sugar, is something you can do on a physiological level, which can help better your relationship with food and help you find freedom from food anxiety. When you spend less energy thinking about food, you can devote more energy to those things in life that really matter.

The mental and emotional. This encompasses the mindset shifts you can undergo in order to start thinking about food, health, your body, and yourself in a more positive light. These first two facets have been very influential in developing my philosophy in the first place. Clearly from the nutritional perspective, if you can get out of the calorie-counting mindset (the place rooted in lack, scarcity, restriction) and start viewing food as nutrients, which are represented in your food by different colors, you can start to think of food in a more positive way. As I have already mentioned, it is as if you are using your plate as a canvas and creating a beautiful collage of colors with your food.

The spiritual. The deeper work comes with finding true happiness. You can't just eat real foods, improve your relationship with food, get healthier physically, and expect to be happier from there (although many believe this to be the case). It's not about the food, it's not about your body, and it's not even about your physical health. The emotions you are wanting to feel come with cultivating your spiritual health. Spirituality cannot be separated from the relationship you have with yourself. To connect to your true, authentic self is one of life's greatest gifts.

When I stopped attaching who I was to my physical body, I was able to step more fully into my authenticity. This was not a one-time occurrence but rather a realization that triggered, and continues to influence, a gradual unfolding. I can attest to the fact that there is nothing more liberating than breaking free from being at war with your body. By tuning in to your intuition and what works for *you*, you will learn to release the external chatter and bombardment of messages that might be creating confusion and standing in the way of your ideal health and most authentic self. When you have this ability in your back pocket, it is always available to you. Even if you veer "off course," you know how to get back to a place that feels good. I encourage you to travel inward—return to yourself and what lights you up. This directional change of focus created the foundation for pursuing and achieving some of my greatest goals and dreams. With a mindset shift toward feeling abundant, counting more color in my life brought a deeper appreciation of what was going well in my life, rather than focusing on the lack or what I needed to fix.

STARTING RIGHT NOW,
WE ARE GOING TO GET REAL!
I HOPE TO GUIDE YOU TOWARD MAKING
A CONNECTION TO WHAT IS REAL
ACROSS VARIOUS REALMS OF HEALTH,
WHILE EXPLORING
THE BALANCE BETWEEN
BODY, MIND, AND SPIRIT.

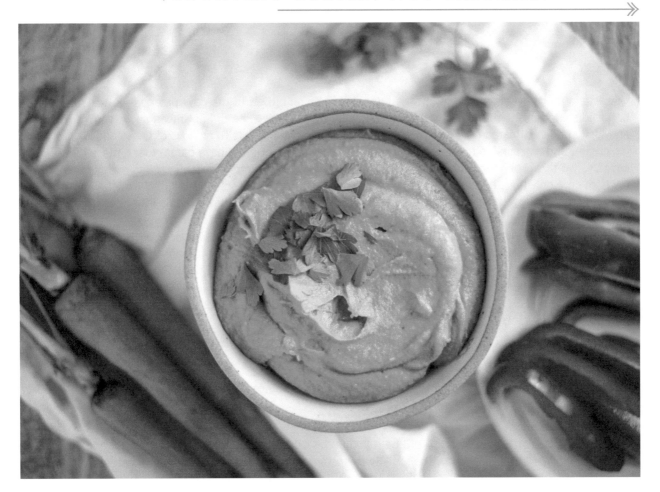

chapter one:

THE INFLUENCE OF STORY

i was about eight years old the first time I decided to go on a diet. In the days preceding, my dad had said something about my weight. To his defense, I truly believe he did not mean any harm and likely underestimated how impressionable young girls can be. Due to my love of Oreos and ice cream, and an aversion to fruits and vegetables, the comment must have come from a place of concern, yet this experience shaped my lens. It is the first time I remember feeling shame about my body; not only that, it planted a seed—a deeply ingrained, subconscious seed about my beliefs, which not only affected the way I saw myself but also influenced my behavior and sense of worth in the world. To clarify, this realization did not occur back then but rather over twenty years later when I was doing a lot of work on myself. I am not referring to physical work; as a health coach and fitness instructor, I felt as if I had that side of myself down to a science. It was the mental and emotional walls of my past that I was attempting to tear down. Through this work, the not-so-pretty memories would resurface. The first time I decided to go on a diet was one of them.

I approached my mom soon after receiving the comment from my father, and our exchange went something like this:

> **Me:** "Mom, I think I need to lose weight. For the next few days,
> I am going to eat nothing but bananas."

> **Mom:** "Oh Sara, if you want to lose weight, bananas are not the way to go,
> they have a lot of sugar."

I know what you might be thinking right now. You are probably gasping in slight horror at my mother's response. If I were you, I would be thinking the same thing: *What kind of mother would say such a thing!? Isn't it a woman's responsibility to nurture and ensure her daughter grows up with a positive body image?*

Absolutely, but please keep in mind that in the 1990s, the campaign to embrace your body no matter the size or shape was not a societal message as it stands today. I hold zero blame. Looking back on it, I am now fully aware she was stuck in her own cycle and body image issues. My mother was always experimenting with different programs and plans, from counting calories to counting points, to Atkins and South Beach, and everything in between. While this is an unfortunate environment for any adolescent girl to be exposed to, I do not think my mother knew any better; for that I feel only compassion.

Tracing my health "story" to its beginning, this memory is where I turn back its pages. I think there are many women who can relate. The dieting mindset is all too pervasive in our culture, and while I believe there has been a general shift in a more positive direction, it persists. If there is anything that does a number on one's relationship with food and self-esteem, it is the restriction mentality that is so closely associated with dieting. This is what I call the scarcity model.

What this experience also taught me was to fear food. Before the conversation with my mom, I believed bananas to be healthy; afterward, I did not want to eat them for fear they were going to make me fat. Little minds are malleable. While this thought process was taking place subconsciously at the time, I learned to categorize certain foods as either good or bad. I learned to place judgement on something that was not inherently moral. I did not unlearn this tendency until my late twenties. For decades, when it came to viewing various foods, I constantly looked through a lens of judgement. When there is judgement attached to something—not to mention something we must have multiple times per day in order to *survive*—we are faced with choices on a daily basis that will then lead to certain emotions.

We feel happiness, joy, and pride when we do (or eat) something good; or guilt, shame, frustration, and fear when we do (or eat) something bad. Eventually, these daily judgements take a toll not only on our relationship with food but also on our emotional health and the way we view ourselves.

Fast-forward a decade down the road to when I was a senior in high school. During that span of time, I was never overly focused on food. Being a happy, growing teen who played sports and was very active, I never even really thought about it. I cared more about boys than my body. My friends used to always point out how I even danced during mealtime. I loved eating! But by the time senior year rolled around, and the previous couple of years were spent snacking while studying, indulging in dessert every day, and experimenting with alcohol (i.e. partying), with no knowledge of nutrition under my belt, the pounds had piled on. Then one day someone made a comment about my weight. Due to my particular story, the comment was more triggering and impactful than it might have been to someone else with a different history. It resurfaced my poor relationship with food and fear of "getting fat," and basically started a downward spiral into serial dieting.

Clinical psychologist Dr. Sue Johnson calls this "rubbing a raw spot." She defines a raw spot as a "hypersensitivity formed by moments in a person's past."[4] While much of her work pertains to relationships—how our attachment needs and the sensitivities that show up in romantic relationships can often be traced to those critical relationships with parents and siblings in our developmental stages—I believe her theory can be loosely applied to my experience. Tara Mohr, leadership coach and author of *Playing Big*, explains that a criticism or insult stings that much more when in congruence with a belief we hold about ourselves, a phenomenon she calls "the matchup."[5] The experience has less to do with what is said but rather strikes a stronger chord when it confirms negative views we hold about ourselves. Research shows I am not alone: It is estimated that 20 to 40 percent of women struggle with body dissatisfaction.[6] Therefore, it seems likely others share a similar story or may be able to pinpoint a similar experience.

College is where things took a compulsive turn. I was terrified of gaining "the freshman fifteen," and was determined not to become another statistic affirming the amount of weight first-year college students typically gain. In all honesty, the avoidance of weight gain was probably a higher priority for me than getting good grades. Thanks to a combination of confusion about what adequate nutrition entailed and a fast-developing eating disorder, I over-exercised and I under-ate. After dropping to a very low weight, despite multiple comments from family and friends, I felt happy and accomplished. It makes me sad to think about that now, and even sadder to think there are others who still feel this way. For me, I now know that it was simply another shiny penny for me to pick up. I will explain more about this in a later chapter, but it ties into one of my long-held beliefs of "not being good enough." Because my sense of self-worth was so low, I needed to win the weight loss game to formally give myself permission to feel *enough*. All of these elements of my experience came crashing together: I was attaching my self-worth to my physical appearance, while simultaneously feeling like a small fish in a big collegiate pond, while *also* trying to make friends for the first time since I was five years old. Understandably, this belief went from an underlying whisper to an obsession.

The "happiness" I felt in response to losing weight, forgoing a feared food, or forcing my body through another gym session was always fleeting, quickly replaced by the intense anxiety of gaining it all back. Over the next four years I "yo-yo dieted" and my weight followed suit. I gained back the original weight I had lost my first year and then some, worsening my relationship with food and my emotional well-being as a result. Not only did I feel out of control (ironically, since control was ultimately what I was seeking), but I could not understand why I did not have the "willpower" to land on and stay at a weight I wanted to be. I now know willpower has nothing to do with it.

If you share a story like mine, or even if you do not to this extreme but have been stuck in a dieting cycle, or even have just been on a diet once and felt like you failed, there is so much more to consider on the mental side of things, especially concerning conditioning, mindsets, and subconscious beliefs. When it comes to weight loss from a purely physiological standpoint, the archaic model of "calories in, calories out" is an over-simplification. Hormones, digestion, and even the more abstract areas of physical health, such as stress and sleep, all play a role. But it is the power of the mind that largely goes overlooked. To some extent, my thoughts, beliefs, and anxieties around my self-image were keeping me rooted in a place I did not want to be because it was something I was so focused on. The Law of Attraction states that what you focus on you attract, and I strongly believe this phenomenon was playing out in my experience. I will explain more about the Law of Attraction and the power of the mind in later chapters.

After college, my eating conditions stabilized a bit. I discovered healthy-living blogs and felt inspired by others who had adopted a more balanced approach to food and exercise. I educated myself more on nutritional science and started to get more creative in the kitchen. My weight was more consistent, and inner shifts were being made. Not only did I start to look at food more objectively but I also started to make the connection between what I ate and how I felt, both physically and emotionally. Prior to this point, eating had always been attached to what I looked like and the number that would show up on the scale. Now I was learning more about the medicinal power of eating more plants and how inflammatory foods, such as sugar, negatively impact my mental health.

Please know that it is not as if big, sweeping changes happened overnight. Even though I was making strides, I was still struggling with releasing my anxiety around food and exercise. At this point, I was in my mid-twenties and was simultaneously going through some tough personal things pertaining to family, career, and romantic relationships. I felt quite lost and lacked passion and purpose. I found myself in a frequent state of victimhood (another psychological tendency I picked up along the way, which is another story for a different day), leaving me feeling disempowered and depressed. My views on health and on myself were improving, yet the fear and need to control were still present, given the lack of control I felt in other areas of my life. There remained a compulsion for food—a constant worrying about where my next meal was coming from, wondering whether I was actually physically hungry, and if so, would I have healthy options available. Fundamentally, there was a lack of self-trust and an inability to be fully present. Food anxiety, which I define as thinking and worrying about food when it is not there in front of you, is a prime example of being stuck in the past or propelled into the future. There was also this underlying belief that if I could just figure it out, fit my way of eating into a pretty box and tie it beautifully with a bow, I would finally be happy. Again, just another lie I (i.e. my ego) was telling myself.

Not only is this perception painstakingly wrong, but there are so many pieces to unpack. It is obvious to me now that the relationship I had with food mirrored the relationship I had with myself. On the outside, I may have appeared to be a happy twenty-something girl who was thriving, but internally, I felt like I was failing to find my footing in life. The fact that I was in my mid-twenties and felt as if I needed to have my life figured out says more about our society than it does about me. Therefore, I clung to food and physical activity, as these were the areas I could control. Only I was not in control—I was caught in a cycle characterized by self-judgement of being "good" versus "bad" with my eating and exercise. Monday through Friday I would restrict my caloric intake and hold myself to a regimented exercise schedule; during the weekends, I would become unhinged. I would over-compensate with an over-consumption of alcohol, and in my intoxicated state I would binge eat. Never once did I think there was a root issue pertaining to my subconscious thoughts, behaviors, and beliefs. I thought the solution was found on the surface: That if I could just stop overeating, everything would be right in my world. I ignored the dark emotions swirling underneath, and the cycle kept spinning. In hindsight, I can see why I was choosing to stay in it—this cycle served as a safety blanket.

The Cycle as a Safety Blanket

Although being caught in this cycle did not *feel* safe at the time, ironically, it served as a distraction from the negative emotions I was feeling on a deeper level. These emotions were ones that I was both conscious of and those that were buried in my subconscious. It was "easier" to pinpoint the food and exercise issues as the source of my unhappiness, and what I (mis)perceived wrong with my body, than it was to acknowledge and hold space for what felt too big and burdensome to bear. Because my mental energy was preoccupied with the physical, it numbed the negativity taking place in the more emotional and spiritual aspects of my life. The sense of achievement from "getting back on track" allowed me to feel happy and gave my human brain something to fix, even if the feeling was ephemeral and solution unsustainable.

In her book Women, *Food and God*, Geneen Roth describes compulsive eating as "a way we leave ourselves when life gets hard...[it] is a way we distance ourselves from the way things are when they are not how we want them to be...ending the obsession with food is all about the capacity to stay in the present moment."[7] Roth goes on to state that the obsession with food (such as mine) gives you something to do, something surface-level to focus on in the face of "heart-shattering" and heavy life stuff. She compares this mental game to "Sisyphus pushing the boulder up the mountain." As long as your mind is preoccupied with eating (something we must do multiple times a day), body image and weight, and the sense of achievement attached to the occasional achievement of goals (the number on the scale, preparing the "perfect" meal, the workout ticked off the to-do list), there will always be something to work toward. Having a tendency toward perfectionism, my type-A personality wrapped this addiction to food and weight around me like a comforting cloak, shielding me from the loneliness, anger, and insecurity that arose if my mind became too still.

In his book *The Mindbody Prescription*, Dr. John Sarno describes this tendency as a "defense mechanism," a way in which the mind and body work together when there are difficult repressed emotions in one's subconscious.[8] The diversion of one's attention to the physical body allows for the avoidance of negative feelings. I believe this can manifest in a number of different ways. While Dr. Sarno speaks more to actual physical symptoms (back pain, stomach problems, and skin issues to name a few, all three showing up in my story as well), the fixation on the body with regard to disordered eating and over-exercise is another example.

Finding Freedom from the Cycle

So how did I break free from this cycle? Some major shifts occurred in my late-twenties and early-thirties that allowed me to not only view food and health in a completely different light (neutral and objective at first, positive and loving shortly thereafter) but to also start to develop a more positive and loving relationship with myself through the inner work I referenced earlier; again, not just with my physical health but the essence of who I am. I also learned to forgive my past and the choices I made that put me on this path. I did not go at this alone but rather with the help of therapists, my amazing life coach, and my loving partner, who eventually became my husband. As I write these words, I feel grateful for the unfolding of my story; it has influenced the person I have become. Although it took me decades to declare it, I love who I have become.

This inner work is powerful and what I have come to realize as one of life's greatest gifts. I will go deeper into how you can incorporate inner work and self-awareness into your life, but know that the relationship you have with yourself is the most important relationship there is; it is the avenue to inner peace. When you can be your own best friend, feeling lost or alone simply can't exist; you will always feel supported. I was recently listening to a podcast on self-love, and the host asked her audience if they had ever held their own hand, a gesture that many do not know. But I was able to nod my head in affirmation. In fact, there have been many times, whether in meditation, yoga class, or sitting still with sadness and grief, when I have done just that. I have loved ones I can easily reach out to, but sometimes the reassurance from yourself that everything will be OK is one of the strongest signs of healing.

I argue that when it comes to changing something about yourself, whether in the realm of body, behavior, belief, all three, or something else entirely, self-love is the foundation for making that change sustainable. For me, a lack of self-love was the missing piece through those years of turmoil, and my habits and behaviors reflected it. Think about it: If you do not love your body, you are not really going to care how you treat it. Think about something else you don't like: an old sweatshirt or an ugly piece of furniture. Without respect, there is no holding these things in high regard. Furthermore, when there is a deviation from your intuition—that inner sense of peace in your heart—this chasm creates quite the feeling of discomfort and increases the likelihood that you might engage in some self-destructive behaviors.

If you feel that you have a good relationship with yourself, I hope you celebrate that! You may be much further along than many women out there. Even if this is where you are, I hope you hang tight, as I still firmly believe you will learn something in the subsequent chapters. We will explore mindful eating (which we all need reminders of), mindfulness in general, consciousness, energy, presence, vibration, and flow. I encourage you to stay open and, at a minimum, engage in some self-reflection. This is a journey of getting real; a balance of nutritional science, holistic health, and mindset shifts. Real food and real you—not to mention that the present moment is the only thing that is real.

The Role of Trauma

Before I move on, I find it important to address the role of trauma. When I was in my mid-twenties, sitting in a chair opposite my therapist, an experience from my early childhood slowly bubbled to the surface through flashbacks and a gradual uncovering of distant memories. I had repressed this physical trauma for over two decades. While acknowledging it and then having to talk about it was far from easy, it shed light on so much. I'll be honest, even though accepting this aspect of myself lifted something off my shoulders that had been weighing me down, I still felt shame around it for years. Not only did I hide it from my closest loved ones, but every time the trauma came to mind, I quickly pushed it away.

It has only been in my thirties, as I continue to do some deep inner work around my trauma, that it has finally started to lose its grip. I can view it with more objectivity and neutrality; as something that is a part of my story instead of something that happened "to me." To look at it as the latter would keep me feeling victimized by it. I have come to a place where I have wanted to take my power back. I was done feeling shame and sick of feeling small. I can now more openly consider it as what "was" and what "is" without the self-judgement of shame. Doing so has not only been liberating but has also allowed me to receive more insight into the *why* behind certain limiting (i.e. destructive) beliefs and mindsets.

For example, I believe underneath my desire to be thin, and my former obsession with weight loss, food, and fitness, was the underlying need to feel free in my body—to feel comfortable and confident versus the heavy burden of this negative experience. This makes total sense to me, and with this understanding comes acceptance. My trauma made me feel so out of control; physically at the time, and mentally and emotionally in the aftermath, even if subconsciously. Food and anything to do with my physical body and health were simply other ways to control what I could. The difference between how I operated when these memories were subconscious versus bringing them to light has everything to do with awareness. Consciousness not only for the trauma but also for the behavior as a result, has simply lessened the anxious energy surrounding this side of myself. I can compartmentalize and return to the present reality without running on old programming. I will be completely honest: The desire to feel light energized in my body remains; in fact, I believe everyone deserves to feel that way physically. I still exercise almost every day and eat in a way that makes me feel energized and clear-headed. Yet it is not tied to a compulsory need but rather has been replaced by a loving sense of self-care and compassion. From that place, it makes my journey with health more pleasant.

This is an example of "story" that might fall on the extreme end of the spectrum, but it is one I know exists for many others. First understanding you are not alone can be empowering and lighten the load. If you are able, you too can engage in some inner work around your experience, either alone or with a trained professional. Whether this resonates with you or not, I encourage you to take some time to journal about your individual story, specifically as it pertains to your health.

journal:

What has your path been like up to this point? Write down whatever flows without attaching too strongly to it or judging yourself for the way things have been. It is your story, so it will never be erased, but just because this is the way things have been, does not mean it is the way things will have to be. Putting pen to paper can be a powerful tool and may help you look at your past with a bit more objectivity or with compassion and forgiveness, if that applies.

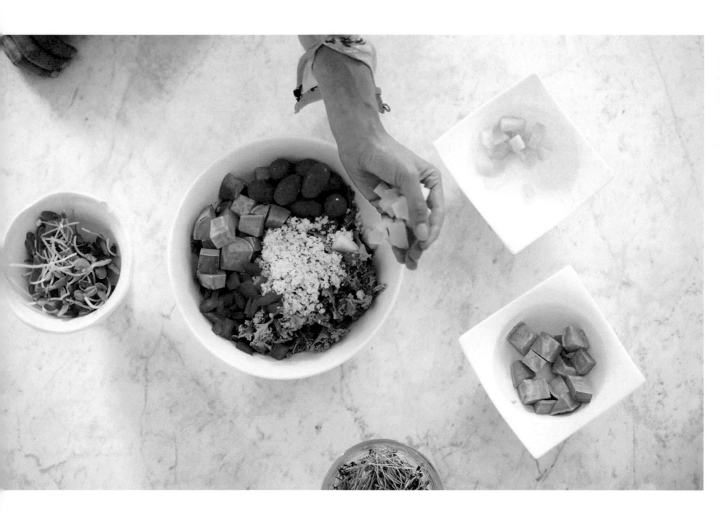

chapter two:

A New Model of Thinking and Believing

*b*efore we go over the nitty-gritty nutritional science in the next chapter, I want to introduce a game-changing idea to help you shift your belief system about the attachment of emotions to outcomes. This is particularly relevant if my story resonated with you, and can be applied to anything you want, whether that pertains to your physical health or something else entirely.

You see, because weight loss was often talked about in my household, I was conditioned to believe that it was something that *mattered*. The message was that as a woman, being on a diet was something I should prioritize. My mother never sat me down and said these words, but just by watching, observing, and listening, I absorbed this to be true. And my perceptions around all of it from a very early age were far from positive. Furthermore, I learned that not only did it matter but it was also a prerequisite to perceiving yourself positively.

There's the rub, and it is something I want you to realize: Your mindset around something is going to affect how you perceive it, and your perception is going to affect your experience. Someone who grew up in an environment where food, dieting, and weight were rarely talked about, or better yet, someone who was taught to embrace a positive body image and love themselves no matter their size, shape, or number on the scale, is going to have had a completely different system of thoughts, emotions, and beliefs instilled in them.

No matter if you find yourself in the former camp or not, the amazing thing about awareness is that each moment offers you an opportunity to choose. It is easy to play victim to the stories of our pasts, but growth comes as a result of taking responsibility for our thoughts and emotions *now*. This life presents us with many things we cannot control, but our thoughts and the way we respond to external circumstances are both in the realm of what we *can* control.

Brook Castillo, CEO and co-founder of The Life Coach School, teaches that when we have a thought, whether about a circumstance or something in our experience, "that thought is always going to create a feeling. The feeling is always going to create an action, an inaction, or a reaction. That action will create a result."[9] Once I heard this new paradigm, it completely changed my perspective from the old model of how I walked through life, waiting for the next shiny penny to pick up; it was backward from how I had always operated. I was raised to believe happiness came as a result of achieving something: the grades, the job, the body, the boyfriend, the attention. But even after the obtaining or achieving, the resulting "happiness" is not often sustainable. Without awareness for what is taking place, and the establishment of a fundamental sense of security, the ego will simply find something else to focus on. The human brain will laser in on another goal to obtain before one can feel fulfilled.

In her book *Super Attractor*, spiritual teacher Gabby Bernstein affirms this mindset as a result of societal conditioning: "We've been waiting for life's circumstances to give us a reason to feel good. In fact, many of us don't realize that it is a decision we've made...When we do this, we're putting the outcome before the feeling. We have it all twisted!"[10] It is an unfortunate cultural phenomenon that we are raised to think this way. We are swinging from one vine to the next in this jungle of life, thinking that achieving something outside of ourselves is a prerequisite to being happy; this simply sets us up for emotional failure. Multiple research studies on positive psychology and neuroscience affirm that this belief system has it all wrong. Author and happiness researcher Shawn Achor emphasizes that when working to attain a goal, feeling happy first increases the likelihood for success, not the other way around.[11]

The archaic model is exactly what the dieting industry tries to sell: happiness—that weight loss must come first before we can feel the desired emotion. If you are still counting calories or approaching your physical health from a place of anxiety, I urge you to try something different. In every health coaching consultation I hold with my clients, I have them reflect on their health goals. After digging deeper, I discover that even if the goal initially sounded more physical (a certain number on the scale, more muscle definition, increased energy), the work became more about the way they would eventually *feel* after achieving the goal: vibrant, confident, happy, free. Most of the time, however, my clients' experiences with their health and bodies up to the point they walk through my door share similar aspects of my story. Their path has been permeated with suffering and stress. The Law of Attraction emphasizes that it is not likely you will achieve sustainable happiness at the end of a journey laced with negative emotion. I will get more into the Law of Attraction in a later chapter.

What if we flip the script? What would happen if you started with feeling the positive emotions *first*? Using the power of choice, we have that ability. The beautiful thing about this process is that it can be applied to anything in life. Begin with what you want, reflect on the desired feeling you will feel after obtaining or achieving it, and embrace it now—let go of the rest. This is the Law of Attraction; this is getting into a flow and expanding your energy to attract the result you have been searching for all along.

Trust me, I know—easier said than done. That is why I am going to walk you through actionable steps you can take to make this happen. Positive affirmations, journaling exercises, mindset shifts, and your greatest tool of all: your physical body. That's right, the very thing you may have been resenting all along will become your greatest asset. As humans and energetic beings, emotions are literally felt in the body. My life coach and mentor introduced me to "The Body Compass" and it is something I turn to daily. Not only can it help you tap into those elusive emotions but it can also help you make decisions. I will dive more into this in later chapters.

journal:

I encourage you to pause here and reflect. Read over your health story you previously wrote, and journal about the emotions you have been wanting to feel. Then ask yourself: What can you do or say to yourself to feel them now? This is the power of positive affirmations. Additionally, think about a time in your past when you felt vibrant/energized/joyful. Describe how that felt in your body. Then start to embrace those sensations now. Cultivating a positive inner environment first has amazing implications for both your physical and emotional health.

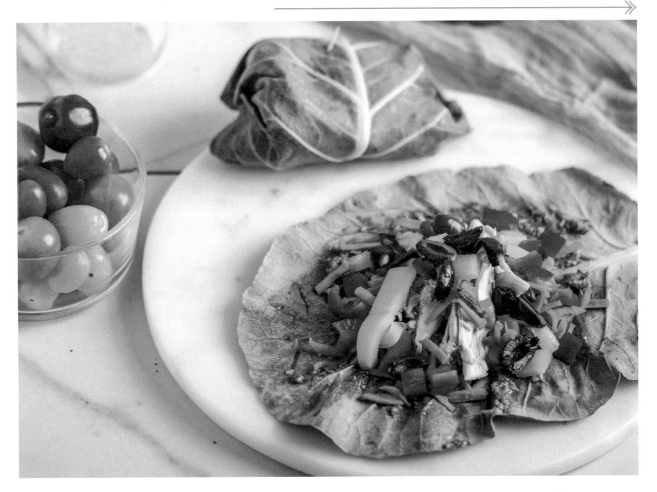

chapter three:

Upshifting to Neutrality with Nutritional Science

*I*f you have had a fearful relationship with food up to this point, learning the nutritional science behind metabolism, hormones, and how our bodies work—while shifting away from the archaic dieting model of calories in, calories out—is an empowering next step. Information is power, and discovering what weight loss and maintenance entails can enable you to make better-informed choices from a place of objectivity.

As you have read, I grew up with the notion that weight loss was all about eat less, move more. The way our bodies work is not so black and white. Our metabolism operates as more of a chemistry lab than a calculator. The processes that take place after eating are much more complex. Hormones, stress, sleep, and, yes, your emotions, all play a part.

There is an abundant amount of information when it comes to the "right way" to eat, which creates a lot of confusion. As soon as one dietary theory gets touted as being the end-all-be-all for attaining better health, another one replaces it; this leads to a lot of uncertainty and fear around food in and of itself. People are so used to looking outside of themselves for answers and quick fixes that they lose the connection to themselves and what works for their individual bodies. Turning to your own awareness and intuition will also be important because bio-individuality must be factored in. In other words, what works for one person is not going to work for the next. Every body is unique and different, so one's way of eating should be as well. Then you must take into consideration that every day is different, with its individual demands. Depending on what someone has going on, how much he or she slept the night before, where she is in her menstrual cycle, or the amount of stress he or she is feeling, there is no way a blanket approach to nutrition seems reasonable. The more you turn inward, listen to what your body wants and needs, and *know thyself*, the more you set yourself up for success.

But for right now, we are going to practice the art of non-judgement. For example, in consideration of calorie counting, a "calorie" becomes something we try to restrict, thereby judging it as "bad" as a result. From a societal perspective, I do believe people are moving in the right direction with health, shifting away from calorie counting and understanding that there is more to it than that, but I still hear about calorie counting from my health coaching clients, so I know it persists.

Let's practice: What objectively is a calorie? A calorie is simply a unit of measurement of the energy potential of the foods we eat. There are foods that have more energy potential than others. Categorizing foods in their respective macronutrients, fat contains nine calories per gram and carbohydrates and protein contain about four calories per gram. Unfortunately, this is why "fat" gets such a bad rap, because everything else being equal, fat contains more calories per gram. Again, it's not so black and white, and I even view this as a good thing because eating high-quality sources of fat will energize, fuel, and satiate you more than other foods.

When you understand that food is *information for your cells*, you begin to embrace a truth for what is and release the emotional fear around it. To oversimplify, whenever you eat, the food travels through your digestive tract, nutrients get absorbed in your small intestine, sent into your blood stream and then to your cells, with the rest getting discarded as waste. Simultaneously, many hormonal reactions take place, signaling your body to undergo certain physiological processes.

Nutrition and fitness expert Mark Sisson explains that "every bite of food is a hormonal experience." Thinking about eating in this way, and considering how your body may react to the food you put in, can help motivate your choices. Mealtime becomes more than just ingesting calories. It also explains why you cannot exercise away a bad diet or binge from the evening before; internally, there is so much more to it. Understanding the role that blood sugar management—or what I call the *beauty of blood sugar balance*—plays in the eating process can help shed some light on the intricate system of hunger hormones.

The Beauty of Blood Sugar Balance

When I learned more about blood sugar, hunger hormones, and digestion, and the role these elements play in the eating process, I was able to release the dieting mentality that had plagued me for years.

For example, whenever you eat a carbohydrate, no matter if it is a baked good or Brussel sprout, it gets broken down to glucose, another name for sugar in its simplest form. As a response, your pancreas releases the hormone insulin to gather the glucose and send it to your cells for energy. The first three places this glucose travels to are your brain, muscles, and liver; however, the space in your muscles and liver is limited, with a total storage capacity of about 400 and 100 grams respectively.[12] Therefore, excess glucose gets transported to your liver, converted to triglycerides (i.e. fat), and stored in your adipose tissue (i.e. fat cells), where the capacity is *unlimited*. If you have been fearing dietary fat to this point, understanding that eating dietary fat exclusively does not lead to weight gain should be very liberating! Thankfully, research is revealing how beneficial healthy forms of dietary fat are to our physical and mental health, and that excess glucose—or sugar—is the culprit behind many health issues, from metabolic disorders to diabetes to other forms of chronic disease.

When I more fully understood the science behind what went on *in the body* when I ate, the information freed me from food anxiety and dieting. It helped me to release my fear and get back to what is true. After shedding the layers of confusion and fear, I was able to take a more neutral stance around food and nutrition. I then began to view my body more positively as well. Rather than seeing it as something to pick apart and criticize, I came to view it as a smart and efficient machine that was simply doing its job. This perspective was an improvement from the body image issues I had always struggled with.

The work I did on myself eventually evolved to something deeper, something more spiritual. You might have heard the quote, "We are spiritual beings having a human experience," and this message improved my relationship even further. I began to see my body as something on my side—a vehicle with which I move through life. Again, this shift did not occur overnight; for me, the progression moved from negativity to neutrality first.

Physiologically, your body is always working to get back into balance. When you eat, certain hormones are released to achieve a state of homeostasis. Insulin is a major one to keep in mind and is known as your storage hormone, as its role is to shuttle nutrients that aren't immediately needed for fuel to be stored. Given that your hormones are all chemical messengers sending certain signals to brain and body, the presence of insulin in the blood signals to the body that there is glucose (i.e. sugar) circulating.

Should weight loss be one of your goals, this information is important to know. In my health coaching practice, when women come to me to lose weight, I talk about it in terms of *fat* loss because to burn fat more efficiently without losing muscle is ultimately the goal. While this book is not specifically tailored to be a fat-loss program, I believe understanding how our bodies work and the role that hormones play in the process can help clear some confusion, prevent calorie counting, and encourage you to take more of an objective rather than anxious view on the matter.

Hormones play a large role in lipolysis, or the breaking down of stored body fat; therefore, it is important they are balanced and able to do their job. Managing blood sugar is key in balancing hormones, because if you were to think of your hormonal system like a symphony, insulin and leptin (the two hormones most associated with balanced blood sugar) are basically like the conductors. When they are off, the whole song is going to seem wrong.

Hormones are chemical messengers, so in order for your body's fat cells to release stored body fat, they must receive the signal from your hormones to do so. Then oxidation must occur, which entails the released body fat traveling through the blood stream, being received by the target cell, and then burned. As you are starting to realize, this process is not so black and white; it is more complex than the calories in, calories out, move more, eat less, theories you may have previously been beholden to.

Your body has two main sources of fuel: glucose and ketones. The former is sugar, and the latter is a byproduct of broken-down stored body fat. The presence of insulin takes your body out of "fat burning" and into "fat storage" mode in a number of ways. If you have just eaten, and your body is actively breaking down carbohydrates, insulin signals to your body that there is glucose present. Insulin also suppresses the hormone glucagon, which is responsible for breaking down glycogen (i.e. stored sugar) from the stores in your muscles and liver in order to be used for fuel. If this hormone is suppressed, then glycogen stores stay full, and more stored sugar increases the likelihood that any glucose floating around will have to be converted to triglycerides and stored as fat in your adipose tissue. Additionally, elevated levels of insulin suppress the hormone-sensitive lipase (HSL) enzyme, which is responsible for breaking down and releasing fat.[13]

Lastly, the hormone estrogen as well as thyroid function also play roles in the fat-burning process. There are certain receptors found on the surface of your cells that bind with certain hormones to either slow fat loss or speed it up; excess estrogen slows it down, while the thyroid hormone speeds it up. This is why it's important to have your thyroid functioning properly and another reason why stress (which taxes your adrenal glands and therefore impacts your thyroid hormone) can inhibit fat loss.

Stress plays such a larger role than people give it credit for, and I will go into more detail about stress and the hormone cortisol in the next chapter. The major takeaway here is that your hormones are delicate, and to balance them is a complicated thing. Blood sugar balance helps to ensure that the two major hormones, insulin and leptin, are moderated and working adequately so they can do their job efficiently. The food you eat majorly affects these two key players in a significant way.

My goal for providing you with this nutritional science is to have you stress *less*; to not only have you look at your beliefs and stories but also to increase your motivation for eating more real, colorful food. To consume the food that nature intended nourishes your body while supporting blood sugar management and hormonal balance.

It is also important to point out the pervasive myth in the nutrition world that encourages eating smaller meals or snacking throughout the day to keep your metabolism stoked and to burn fat. I want to reiterate here that everyone is different, so if this rhythm of eating works for you, please do not let me influence you otherwise. However, the multiple meals per day structure goes against blood sugar balance and what fat burning entails. While carbohydrates elicit a larger insulin response than protein and fat, insulin *is* released every time you eat, which is a good and natural thing; insulin is our storage hormone after all, and we need nutrients from all foods to be stored. The issue arises when our bodies stay in storage mode and then become desensitized to insulin's message.

Given that insulin is responsible for ushering glucose to our cells from energy, if your cells no longer respond, glucose remains in the blood stream, blood sugar stays elevated, and this creates a hormonal cocktail for chaos. The dysregulation of insulin has negative implications for other key chemical messengers (such as glucagon and leptin) that play a big role in blood sugar balance as well. Furthermore, if you are eating too frequently, this could be impacting your energy. Digestion is a very taxing and labor-intensive process, so if you are eating every two to three hours, you are basically asking your body to undergo a process when it might not have completed the digestive cycle from your previous meal; as a result, your energy can suffer. When you practice the principles of blood sugar balance, you will feel more satiated immediately after and in between meals;[14] this will naturally extend the time between each meal. You will learn in the next chapter how the stress hormone cortisol factors in, which is not only triggered by external circumstances that lead to feelings of fight or flight but even by the thoughts you think. All the more reason we can't minimize health and weight-loss efforts to the calculation of a caloric equation.

This just scratches the surface of blood sugar balance. To learn more, please visit my online course: **www.balancedbloodsugar.com**.

For right now (and going forward), I want you to consider the *quality* of your food. The Standard American Diet consists of a lot of carbohydrate-rich, sugar-laden foods. When you eat a primarily S.A.D. diet (an appropriate acronym), you will notice a lot of brown and white on your plate, and not a lot of color: cookies, cake, bread, cereals, hamburgers, French fries, and even those foods that are marketed to be healthy: sugary energy bars, granola, yogurt. These are the foods your body digests quickly, which instigates that blood sugar spike and crash cycle, leading to issues such as increased hunger and cravings, mood irritability, and low energy. There are low-vibrational foods and high-vibrational foods, and I would put processed foods found in the Standard American Diet into the former. Blood sugar mismanagement not only negatively effects weight but also causes symptoms such as brain fog, fatigue, and irritability.

Creating a plate with more colorful options—*real*, whole food—can help you feel clear, energized, and vibrant so you can feel more connected to your better self and spirit; more connected to your essence. When you eat more colorful food found in nature, your brain and body feel fueled, nourished, and clear. As a result, you become less anxiously attached to your physical body and more emotionally empowered to focus on the aspects of life that matter.

Counting colors *not* calories is a philosophy that embodies this shift to real food, moving through a place of neutrality with the nutritional science to embracing a more positive relationship with it. Food should be a beautiful aspect of our lives; eating is what gives us energy and allows us to live our lives in the first place. Nutrition should not be something that is vilified, over-complicated, or a source of stress. Food is intended to serve a purpose of benefiting your body and even healing when needed. Every time you make a meal, ask yourself: *How is my food benefitting my body? How is my food nourishing my mind? How is my food serving my spirit?* It does so in the form of nutrients, represented by the various colors found in fruits, vegetables, other plant-based foods, and high-quality proteins. As you start to eat more real, you will notice more color on your plate.

Let me insert a disclaimer here: Shifting to a more whole foods diet is not about perfection. There are times in life when we will eat something more processed, packaged, or a sugary dessert devoid of nutrition. Furthermore, our lifestyles will sometimes necessitate we turn to convenience food, whether we are on-the-go, traveling, or having a particularly busy day. That is completely fine! I even started my natural foods company, Gratisfied, for this very reason. All it takes is a mindset shift so you can meet these moments with neutrality, compassion, and even enjoyment. For example, whereas whole foods nourish your cells, enjoying a piece of birthday cake with loved ones nourishes your *soul*. The way you approach these experiences is what matters, and as long as you savor peacefully, your body will respond in a more positive way than if you were to eat under the umbrella of judgement and guilt. That's right—our emotions affect our metabolism. I will explain more about this in the next chapter.

Consider how you can add in more nutrition. Where in your meals can you incorporate more color? Start to phase out those less-nutritious, processed, and packaged foods with whole, real foods, which are foods that contain one ingredient. Your body knows exactly what to do with the nutrients in apples, almonds, spinach, or sweet potatoes. The majority of processed foods on the market contain ingredients that *you* can't even read, understand, or pronounce. If that is the case, how do you expect your body to understand what you are ingesting?

If you are already very conscious of your nutritional intake, still ask yourself where you can *add* in or incorporate more variety. Try not to think in terms of taking out or removing foods, which leads to a scarcity mindset. Perhaps you can experiment with produce you don't cook with very often. Think seasonally and shop at your local farmers market, picking a fruit or vegetable that is new to you. Play around with different foods. Your plate is your canvas. Create more beauty!

Lastly, where can you let go? Where are you overly judgmental of your food choices? How can you release the fear, rules, and restriction? Food is nothing to be fearful of. As you practice bringing your attention to what is real in the present moment, you will come to appreciate food for its taste, texture, sight, and smell. Whenever you fear a food, you are creating stories around your experience that are likely not true in that moment. A little later, I will discuss more about detaching from these stories and enjoying mealtime for the sensory experience it is, eventually moving past your five senses to how your emotions and thoughts play a role as well.

When I was caught in a cycle of restriction and calorie counting, not only was I emotionally miserable, but I felt as if I was at the mercy of my cravings. I did not know it at the time, but I was highly addicted to sugar; not traditional sweets as you may think (cookies, candy, and cake) but *glucose*. My diet was largely comprised of the types of foods I had been raised on: higher carb, higher sugar, fat-free type foods, which was simply in alignment with the USDA food pyramid and what we were taught was "healthy" (remember the recommendation to eat eight to eleven servings of whole grains?). As I emerged into adulthood and could make my own decisions about what I consumed, I continued to turn to the items marketed as "healthy"—those white and brown colored processed foods that come in a package. When I was so consumed with calorie counting, I wanted to ensure I could add up everything I had eaten as easily as possible. Until I was taught what to look out for, and how to properly read labels (i.e. the list of ingredients, not the number of calories), the majority of the foods I ate came in a box or bag and were also loaded with sugar. Sure, I ate salads from time to time and loved my pre-workout apple slices, but most of my meals were not what I consider the real food I mostly consume today.

You have likely heard the nutritional advice to shop around the periphery of your grocery store, avoiding the inner aisles; the former showcases those one-ingredient produce options, with the latter containing those sugar-laden packaged foods. I was doing the exact opposite, primarily purchasing those brands promoting weight loss. As long as my bread, cereal, and whole grain pasta were high in fiber and low in fat, I was good to go.

It took me years to realize that the brands behind these foods are smart (and I would argue also corrupt). They know they can prey on body image insecurities and manipulate consumer behavior since so many people are confused about what good nutrition and weight loss even entails. They sell the belief that their products can help you achieve the results you are looking for.

While there are health-conscious companies coming on the scene, many food manufacturers care more about their bottom line than they do about the health of the public. Their goal is to maximize profits and keep you coming back for more. By incorporating certain ingredients into their food (think salt, sugar, manufactured fat), they achieve these aims. They know that these highly palatable foods create a cocktail for addiction; not only do they taste good but they also light up the same reward signals in our brains as drugs.[15] Throw in the fact that as humans, our brains are hardwired to crave sweet foods, and, well, it is a pretty difficult spell to break. But again, knowledge is power, and awareness for what is taking place can help you take back control.

Before we move on to the importance of mindful eating, I want to talk a little more about cravings, especially since I think they can be synonymous with the dieting mindset. Often, a reason why someone states they could not stick to a diet is due to the fact that his or her cravings got in the way. When your approach to food is found on a spectrum of extremes, the fact that you "failed" has you sliding to the other end.

Applying the theme of non-judgement, I want you to know that cravings are neither good nor bad; they are present, they exist, and they always will. Cravings are simply a signal, a way your body communicates with you. They are something to be worked with, not something to be fought against. As you shift to a more real food, blood sugar balancing way of eating, cravings will change and become less intense. Refined sugar cravings may decrease, or you may find yourself craving more nutritious foods. But for right now, I want to talk objectively about what they are.

What do I mean when I say cravings are a signal? They are neither random nor negative, meaning just because you have a craving for a certain food (even if it is a non-nutritious food) does not mean there is anything "wrong" with you, and it certainly doesn't insinuate a lack of willpower. You might have noticed by now there can be a spectrum of intensity with your cravings: on one end a whisper, and on the other end something so fierce you can't help but give in; the latter may lead to those uncontrollable feelings in the face of food. Throw in the fact that the mind plays a role in the digestive process (called the cephalic phase of digestion, which I will explain more about), and you could be standing in a bakery, looking at a cookie or piece of cake, and suddenly find yourself walking away with dessert, even though you had no intention of buying anything.

Think about the type of foods our society is bombarded with on a daily basis, whether through media messages, or the mere presence of processed and packaged foods in stores and display cases: the cephalic phase of digestion is constantly triggered. Not only that, but due to the way we were conditioned to eat, most Americans believe these are the foods they should be consuming. Because refined carbohydrate, sugary foods create reward signals in the human brain, when someone eats these foods, they feel happy, whether he or she realizes it or not. The conditioning continues, and without a conscious attempt to rewire the behavior, it becomes habit.

The "benefits" of eating this way are not physical but rather primarily mental, as these foods lack nutrition and, therefore, are not what your body needs. For some people, there is also an emotional component—eating certain foods and satisfying cravings in order to fill an emotional void—which has to do with something deeper. For example, certain foods may be tied to nostalgia, and eating them is an attempt to feel the emotions the memory evokes. Or perhaps the chemical makeup of the food coupled with the act of eating provides a numbing mechanism for life's trials and tribulations. The emotional side to the behavior must be dealt with through exploration of the root of the issue.

What can help further understanding and healing is knowing what is taking place from a biological and biochemical perspective; this is why I encourage viewing cravings more objectively. As a human, you will continue to have cravings, but the trick is to tune in, listen to the signals your body is sending you, and then respond in a nutritious way, *if* you are needing to respond with food at all. Remember, your body is a very smart and efficient machine, always trying to get back into balance. Cravings are an attempt to reach homeostasis if something is off.

For simplicity's sake, I like to categorize cravings into two camps: savory and sweet.

Physiologically, we need sodium for survival, as it's an important mineral for adrenal and thyroid function. When we crave savory foods, sometimes it means we are stressed, our adrenals are taxed, and we are needing sodium for homeostasis. What is a nutritious way to satisfy a savory craving? Try incorporating more high-quality Himalayan sea salt when you are roasting vegetables, have hummus or guacamole on hand, or turn to hard-boiled eggs and olives as a snack.

When we crave sweet foods, it is likely our bodies' call for energy. Given that glucose (the chemical makeup of a carbohydrate) is our bodies' natural form of quick fuel, a sudden sweet craving could be brought on by a couple of different things: Perhaps you are tired due to a lack of sleep or a long day.

Many people notice an increased sugar craving specifically in the late afternoon, or what is also known as "the afternoon slump." According to our natural circadian rhythm, we are actually meant to feel a slight dip in energy during the 4–6 p.m. window due to what's happening hormonally. Our stress hormone cortisol (which keeps us alert) starts to decline, while melatonin (our sleep hormone) starts to rise; it is your body's way of signaling you to slow down. While feeling more lethargic during this time is normal, it is not supposed to feel debilitating. Since the tendency of our society is to push through (completing to-do list tasks or taking care of children), we turn to substances (i.e. sugar) to get the job done, when at the root of the issue is a need for rest.

If this resonates with you, I encourage you to tune in. Next time, take a step back, reflect on how you are feeling, and ask yourself some simple questions. For example: "I'm craving something sweet, and I know that it has more to do with my energy needs and hormones than about the box of Girl Scout cookies sitting on my kitchen table. How can I best respond?" Then make an informed choice. When you can work backward from a place of self-care, you empower yourself to take a better course of action. Can you satisfy your sweet tooth in a more nutritious way in the form of fruit or sweet vegetables? Could you be better off with something high in protein and healthy fat instead, which will give you a much more energy-dense option? For a persistent sweet tooth, I love a juicy Medjool date with nut butter and dark-chocolate chips; this choice definitely does the trick. Or maybe what you need is not food-related at all. Maybe you need to lie down, read a book, take a bath, or go for a walk.

Speaking of sweets, I often get asked about eating dessert after dinner, when the cravings hit hard late at night. Let's look at what is likely taking place: Sugar (i.e. glucose) is your body's natural form of quick fuel. If it is close to your bedtime, you do not actually need *food* fuel at this hour, you probably just need to go to sleep. Or perhaps there was a lack of pleasure and mindfulness while eating dinner (more on that in a later chapter), or you are staying awake scrolling social media, being bombarded by images of influencers' food posts. Insta-cravings are real. No wonder you suddenly have a craving for a dark-chocolate chip almond butter brownie! What you really need to do is put down your device.

When it comes to cravings, listen to your body with curiosity and answer its calls from a place of self-care. You and your body are a team with the same end goals: to feel good, energized, and balanced. If you have a history of dieting and poor body image, or even something more serious such as an illness or other health issues, this might be a more difficult concept to grasp. I encourage you to become more of an observer of your cravings, taking them for what they are: information. When we judge them—labeling that urge to eat another donut as "bad," for example—we tend to attach a negative emotion to that judgement (i.e. guilt and shame, even if this occurs subconsciously), which is not doing you any favors. Judgement and the negative emotions that ensue will only increase cortisol, likely compounding the craving and decreasing willpower as a result.

Cravings will come up, and the trick is in how you respond. People stuck in a cycle of dieting, hunger, and cravings often feel a lack of control in association with their efforts. While it might feel like you have no control over the craving itself, how you answer is completely up to you. If you keep telling yourself "I have no willpower," that thought then becomes an ingrained belief, and your experience will unfold to reaffirm that belief. Your thoughts are powerful. Understanding that cravings are a strong yet natural survival instinct can help you feel more empowered. They are simply a signal, and you have the ability to take a step back and observe. How you answer is completely in your control.

Below I have included a short exercise to help you both observe and pinpoint your cravings. If needed, the exercise can help you explore any emotions that may be at the root of your cravings, should they not be purely physiological. You may also download this chart from my website: **www.saramcglothlin.com/counting-colors-material**.

OBSERVE YOUR CRAVINGS

WHAT ARE YOU CRAVING?

salty   sweet

WHAT ARE YOU FEELING?

stressed   anxious   tired   overwhelmed

lonely   bored   sad   guilty   ashamed

WHAT EMOTION ARE YOU LOOKING TO OBTAIN THROUGH SATISFYING THAT CRAVING?

relief   energy   happiness   joy

amusement   satisfaction   love   excitement

ARE YOU PHYSICALLY HUNGRY?

yes   no

IF YES: WHAT IS A NUTRITIOUS CHOICE THAT WILL SERVE YOU BEST?

IF NO: IS THERE A NON-FOOD-RELATED ACTIVITY YOU COULD CHOOSE INSTEAD THAT WOULD REAP THE SAME EMOTION?

What Stress Has to Do with It

Although I have just scratched the surface, I hope you are beginning to understand that biology, biochemistry, and strong, innate primal programming play a role in your physical experience. To elaborate on survival instincts, it is important to understand a little more about the stress hormone cortisol, which is a key player in the body's stress response. I like to think of our hormones as "chemical messengers," which are responsible for sending certain signals to your brain and body to undergo necessary functions. Cortisol's main message is to get you to fight or flee, but in terms of what this means for your entire endocrine system (having implications for your health and, yes, weight), it is more complex than that. Since there seems to be a strong correlation between dieting, restriction, and food anxiety, there is a good chance that cortisol is showing up more than it is supposed to.

The mind-body connection is very strong. Just like insulin, cortisol exists for a reason: to keep you alive. It is a necessary component for our biological evolution as a species, and yet, in our modern-day society, it's our perception of stress that has garnered its negative reputation, especially when most of us are walking around with chronically elevated levels. According to Gallup's 2018 Global Emotions Report, "people all over the world are more stressed than ever before."[16] Due to our environment, we are not only more stressed more frequently but also viewing this stress as harmful to our health. While studies have shown that stress is tied to higher rates of anxiety, depression, sleep issues, and illness, more research is concluding that one's perception of stress is a key indicator on its effects. In one 2012 study, individuals who reported high degrees of stress *and* perceived that stress to be harmful to their health had higher rates of death compared to those individuals who reported high degrees of stress but perceived it more positively.[17] What is even more interesting is that the latter group had lower mortality rates compared to the group who reported low levels of stress.

In her book *The Upside of Stress*, health psychologist Kelly McGonigal argues that stress is normal, natural, and a positive aspect of our biology.[18] Instead of allowing it to cripple you, use cortisol and stress to your advantage, which was originally nature's intention. As a hormone, cortisol not only helps turn sugar and fat into energy but also improves your body's and brain's ability to use that energy. Our bodies need this chemical messenger for survival in situations of imminent danger but also in less-pressing circumstances when we simply need energy to take action. Stress is something that will never go away; it is built into our biology. When we can change our perception of it, we can use it to our advantage rather than feel as if we need to get rid of it entirely.

Let's examine the role of stress and cortisol from a primal perspective:

If you look at the lives of our primate ancestors, there was no stress in the way we know it today; they hunted, gathered, connected with loved ones, went to sleep with the moon, and awoke with the sun. Stress and anxiety only came about in the face of real danger. It kept them alert and aware in case they needed to fight or flee from a dangerous situation, like a saber-toothed tiger; in other words, it was *acute* stress. Cortisol and stress served our ancestors in situations for survival, and these instincts are very strong. The body and mind connected in a way to keep these early humans alive. As a response to danger, the body needs quick fuel in order to fight the saber-toothed tiger or flee from the situation altogether. Fuel in those days looked very different, coming in the form of plants (fruit, vegetation, nuts, seeds) and animal meat. A midday snack looked more like a handful of berries or a bite of wild boar, not the vending-machine selection from your office break room.

Fast-forward to today, when we live in a world where anxiety-inducing circumstances surround us daily—I would even argue on an hourly basis (or even more frequently if you were to analyze the noise and chatter in your mind, which I will discuss a little later). Every day, stressful situations in our modern society can look like a fellow driver cutting you off on the way to work; your boss yelling at you for an unfinished project; getting into a fight with your spouse; your toddler throwing a tantrum in the middle of a public place; comparing yourself to others on social media; or the constant stimulation from the multitude of text messages and emails. Even if you don't realize it, every time you hear the ding on your phone, it could create a cortisol response. The list goes on. Stress has taken the shape of becoming a *chronic* presence in our lives.

However, our bodies have not biologically evolved to the point where they can discern between danger or death and a fight with a friend that sends us into a stressful state. Everything being equal, it is still a matter of survival. The primary goal of your brain and body is to keep you alive. The response is the same: fight, flee, freeze, and then find food for nutrients needed to (re)fuel. But in our society, with the abundance of processed "convenience" foods, we reach for the fast-digesting, refined carbohydrates, sugar, and other sweets. And get this: Even when there is no fuel in the form of food available, your body has built-in mechanisms to release stored sugar (also known as glycogen) to be released into your bloodstream. Your blood glucose levels can rise *even* if you do not eat, and cortisol creates this response. Either way, your body senses glucose in the blood, and insulin is released by your pancreas. Insulin spikes quickly with the ingestion of sugary carbohydrates or is just present with the elevated blood glucose levels. For those who are dieting, having a hard time losing weight, and walking around with high levels of anxiety and stress, this is important to know because when both cortisol and insulin are elevated, your body is in *ultra* storage mode.[19] These hormones together signal to your body to hold on to other forms of stored fuel (i.e. fat), as you might need the energy later for similar situations of "survival."

Not only do I hope this information provides clarity on how emotions (specifically those on the lower end of the emotional scale, which I will discuss in more detail later) affect you physiologically (cravings, hunger, and hormonal balance), but I also hope it causes you to reflect on your health "story" up until this point. If your approach to better health, whatever that means for you (weight loss, increased energy, or a general sense of wellness), has been laced with stress and anxiety, you must take the effects of cortisol into account. Later in the book, I will make the case that there is a whole other energetic component that you need to consider as well.

If emotional eating is a part of your story, know that negative emotions alone can instigate a stress response. When cortisol increases, blood sugar spikes and then subsequently drops, which can cause you to crave sugar, and the cycle continues. Should you respond with sugar, this creates a hard-to-break feedback loop as sugar lights up reward signals in the brain, resulting in feelings of happiness and pleasure. Your brain remembers the relief it received in this isolated instance, and if repeated enough times, the behavior becomes conditioned, automatically causing you to associate future stress with eating sugar. It is even harder to pinpoint when negative self-talk, poor body image, beating yourself up, guilt, shame, anger, or other harbored emotions from your past are what is causing a stressful inner environment. Have you ever found yourself on autopilot, turning to food to quell a negative emotion, wondering why you don't have the "willpower" to stop? Again, it has nothing to do with willpower; it is biochemistry and our innate survival mechanisms at work.

In a later chapter, I am going to expand on the concept of your inner-dialogue and emotions, and the energetic consequences for your health and self. But bringing it back to mealtime, mindfulness and awareness are so important from a purely digestive standpoint. If you are someone who struggles with digestive issues, such as bloating, gas, constipation, heartburn, or diarrhea, this will be important to pay attention to. While the food you eat affects your digestion, it may not have as much to do with *what* you are eating but *how*.

The body's nervous system has two different states: the sympathetic state and the parasympathetic state. The sympathetic nervous system is the one characterized by the fight or flight response, which kicks into gear and is associated with adrenaline, short, quick breaths, rapid heartbeat, and a need to act. Basically, it is what happens in the face of stress. On the other hand, your parasympathetic nervous system is known as your "rest and digest" response. It feels like slow, deep breathing and a calm heartbeat. It is the state in which your body has a better ability to perform the essential functions to keep everything internal working optimally: digesting food, repairing cells, thinking, creating, planning. As I noted earlier, we are meant to spend most of our time in the latter, and only a short amount of time in the sympathetic state. For many people, this is not the case due to the constant influx of anxiety-inducing circumstances in people's external environment.

What does this all have to do with your eating experience?

A lot of people are eating meals in a sympathetic state: in the car on the way to work, at your desk answering stressful emails, on the couch in front of the TV surrounded by a bombardment of media messages. Even if you are sitting down at a table, alone with your plate of food, it is likely you are looking at your phone, scrolling social media and comparing yourself to others, reading a blog post, or texting with a friend. Trust me, I can be guilty of it too. (I am currently editing this exact paragraph while eating breakfast.) When I am not being mindful, I notice a big difference in how satiated I feel after eating. When distracted, your body can't properly digest and assimilate nutrients.[20] If you are sitting down at a table mindfully eating with family or by yourself, it is likely that it is only for one meal out of the multiple that you eat in a day.

Eating in the face of a stress response, which is easily triggered, does not only have implications for how full you feel; real physical symptoms and maladies can result. According to Marc David, nutritionist, founder of the Psychology of Eating, and author of *The Slow Down Diet*, there are biochemical burdens of eating while under a stressful state. Eating while stressed or anxious means you are in a state of fight or flight; your sympathetic nervous system is activated and digestion shuts down.[21]

One research study defines stress as "a threat to homeostasis," or the internal balance that your body, by way of physiological processes, is always trying to achieve. Being in a state of stress, whether chronically or acutely, impairs interactions between the brain-gut axis and is a contributing factor for multiple gastrointestinal disorders.[22] To name a few: nutrient absorption decreases, good bacteria are destroyed, bowel movement activity slows, insulin resistance heightens, and inflammation increases. Dr. Joe Dispenza, author of *Becoming Supernatural*, states, "When the fight-or-flight nervous system is switched on and stays on because of chronic stress, the body utilizes all of its energy reserves to deal with the constant threat it perceives from the outer environment. Therefore, the body has no energy left in its inner environment for growth and repair, compromising the immune system."[23]

Ailments related to any and all of these issues—leaky gut, low energy, digestive distress, weight gain, and even more serious health issues like chronic disease—could have very little to do with *what* you are eating and more to do with *how*. These symptoms can be quite common given the fact that in our society, the hurried way in which people are consuming food tends to be the norm and not the anomaly. Even when stress is not created from external factors, such as career, relationships, home environment, or physical activity, it could be created from your internal environment: the thoughts that are running through your mind every day.

Has anyone ever asked you about your self-talk? That if you were to speak to your mom or best friend in the same way you speak to yourself, how would that person respond? Or would you never in a million years speak to someone else that way because the things you say to yourself are so cruel and condescending? Be honest with yourself, and if your inner dialogue is primarily negative, know that you could constantly feel under attack. Yes—your self-talk has the ability to send your nervous system into that sympathetic fight-or-flight state of being.

Unfortunately, when experiencing physical symptoms related to the stress connection and mindless meals, many people are unaware and therefore pinpoint the incorrect culprit. Stomach problems? Must be a certain food or, even worse, something to be covered up with medication. Weight gain? Must need to exercise more or choose more punitive forms of high-intensity workouts (which puts even more stress on the body). Low energy? Might need more caffeine. The root of the issue never gets discovered.

If you are suffering from any of these issues, a solution may simply be mindfulness; especially if you are someone who is too hard on yourself, frequently beating yourself up, and engaging in negative self-talk. Realizing that there is not a food, medicine, form of exercise, or even extra hour of sleep that can solve this for you can help you tap into what is truly needed: self-love, compassion, awareness, and alignment with your intuition (when eating and otherwise). I'm going to touch on all of these, but I want to focus on awareness first.

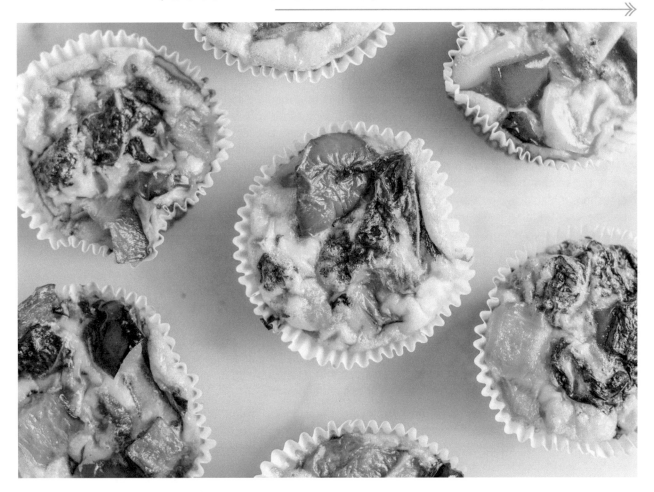

chapter four:

MEALS AS A MICROCOSM OF MINDFULNESS

I define awareness in a couple of different ways: It is that moment-to-moment consciousness that brings you back to the present; then there is also awareness for your awareness, or what I like to call paying attention to your attention. Not only can increased awareness help enhance happiness in your daily life—noticing the small things, so to speak—but it can help you connect to your true self, which is the observer of thoughts, emotions, and energy. I will get more into that later in the book, but when it comes to optimizing your nutrition, awareness is essential to supporting healthy digestion, metabolism, nutrient assimilation, and more. The eating process offers a prime example of being present. Eating is the ultimate sensory experience, a microcosm of mindfulness in our day, but very seldom do we allow ourselves to enjoy it.

Even if you do not have a negative food relationship, people often eat in a distracted state. Layer in the mindsets associated with dieting, restricting, and food anxiety, and you are not only distracted but also likely eating under the grip of the stress response. I have had clients who are not dieting or restricting, per se, but are worried about whether they are eating the "right" foods or exercising the "right" way. They grapple with whether they are doing enough for their health and physical body. Any negative emotions or noisy mental chatter could have the same effect. You have lost the present moment awareness. Furthermore, thinking about food at any time when you are not planning, preparing, or sitting down to eat (which could be a symptom of food anxiety, especially if the thoughts are compulsive) is the epitome of not being present.

Mindfulness is all about that moment of waking up, realizing your mind has wandered off to a place that is not serving you or your present moment, and gently bringing it back. The more you practice, the more you develop the habit. It might never be easy, but it will become easier—that is why it is a practice. As long as we have an active mind (in other words, as long as we are alive), we are always a student in this work. Meditation is a tool to help strengthen your practice, which I will discuss in more detail and encourage later in the book. For right now, I want to reference the eating experience as an example of an active meditation.

While you are eating, you are utilizing most of your five senses: touch, taste, sight, smell. I would argue you utilize hearing as well, if eating alongside company, tuned in to your surroundings, or even just listening to yourself chew. Eating is also what I would call a neutral experience; as a biological need of being human, it is a process we carry out multiple times a day in order to survive. However, if someone has a history of dieting, restricting, disordered eating, and body image issues, there is a likelihood that mealtimes trigger negative emotions—a projection of past "stories," judgement, and associations, leading to layers of complexities and meaning. As a reminder, stories cause us to attach meaning to certain experiences; in this case, eating could be associated with weight gain, loss of control, or a numbing agent. Food and eating, therefore, become subjective.

When you can bring your mind back to neutrality, an acceptance for what is from an objective standpoint, you can start to shift this mindset; in fact, it is a good analogy for anxiety in general. Anxiety can be a self-created construct as a result of thoughts that are stuck in the past or lodged in the future. When it comes to food anxiety specifically, there might be thoughts of past eating experiences or feeling out of control, or thoughts of future fears of foods that won't serve you. I remember when my disordered eating was at its height, I would worry about whether I would have the right snack on hand *hours* later—even when I had just finished my last meal. I was not even hungry, but the anticipation stayed on the forefront of my mind just the same. For me, it was a poor relationship with food exacerbated by blood sugar imbalance. I once had a client describe low blood sugar, the sensation we try to avoid through incessant snacking, and "panic" was the word that came to her mind when describing how she felt in these instances. She elaborated it with a fear of not being able to function. I knew exactly what she meant; it was this very fear that kept me tied to my food anxiety as well. It is why mindful eating, coupled with blood sugar balancing nutrition, can create a strong foundation for food freedom.

In the present moment, whether you are eating or otherwise, when your mind finds stillness, there is just calm, peace, and a realization of what is. There is your breath, your heartbeat, and what you can see and touch right in front of you. Without the negativity, there can only be neutrality. For example, bringing it back to low blood sugar, if you ever found yourself in this state, and subsequently spiraling to the panicked place my client described, you could take a deep breath, feel the sensations in your body, understand that you are hungry, yet you will eat again. You will not pass out and you will not die. Then you take an action step or make a choice to get to a place that feels better. Do you see how that works?

When you do this with your food in general, there is no labeling, judgement, right or wrong, or being "good versus bad;" there is only what is. In this moment, you have the ability to take it a step beyond neutrality to shift upward to positivity. This is a choice you can apply to the food in front of you. To count colors is to start from a mindset of nutritional neutrality, eventually upshifting to more positivity.

Why is this mindset shift important not only for your relationship with food but also for your physical health? I have illustrated the effects of negativity and stress on the eating process, but what about when we eat from a calm, peaceful, positive mindset? When we eat with awareness, pleasure, and enjoyment?

To reiterate, digestion starts in the mind; it is called the cephalic phase of digestion, and it plays a major role in our metabolic process.

A good example of the cephalic phase of digestion at work is when you are watching television. A commercial comes on showcasing a delicious-looking pizza, with melt-in-your-mouth cheese that is oozing off each slice. Your mouth immediately starts to water (it might even be watering right now), and you suddenly think about getting one delivered for dinner. Due to the physiological response of your body from merely seeing this image (salivary glands release saliva and enzymes to jumpstart the digestive process), your brain gets the message that you are now hungry. There is no actual food in front of you, but your brain and body are working in a way as if there is (which is what makes this kind of advertising so effective).

The opposite can also be true: Have you ever been watching television with a bowl of popcorn or bag of chips? It is as if you are eating on autopilot mode, and eventually you look down as your hand swipes an empty space. You realize you have just eaten all the food, yet you could still eat; you still feel physically hungry. This is the absence of the cephalic phase of digestion. Your mind was not present in your eating experience—it did not receive the memo that you just ingested food, hence you do not feel satisfied.

Scientific research supports the importance of the cephalic phase of digestion and the role of the mind during meals, not only in our level of satiety but also in critical aspects of gut function.

In one study, participants were divided into two groups that were both to drink a mineral drink with the aim to test nutrient absorption. The first group was to do so while the researchers spoke into their ears about various topics. The second group was to drink the mineral drink in a calm and relaxed state, concentrating fully on what they were doing. Afterward, they were tested on the absorption rate of the minerals in the small intestine. In the relaxed group, 100 percent of the minerals were absorbed. In the distracted group, 0 percent![24]

Another study looked more closely at digestive activity and gut function. A group of students were to watch a short film, with one subgroup instructed to eat a snack before the film started, while the remainder of the participants were to eat while watching the film. In the former, results showed normal peristalsis, or what are known as digestive contractions (the motion of your gut to keep your food moving along). In the latter, gut motility decreased, and enzymatic secretion dropped, leading them to conclude more inefficient digestion activity while distracted.[25]

These findings have so many implications for your health: decreased nutrient absorption could lead to low energy; less-efficient digestion could lead to gut issues; and a lack of mindfulness may impair metabolism and weight loss or maintenance, while also decreasing feelings of satiety between meals and increasing cravings.

How many of you have been on a diet, or dealt with food anxiety, or simply worried about what you *should* be eating, yet sat peacefully and mindfully with your food, savoring and tasting each bite with pleasure and awareness? I bet this mindset does not create the conditions for an enjoyable eating experience. No, I bet your thoughts are laced with uncertainty and even anxiety from time to time. Maybe you are even denying yourself what you really want, and as a result never feel satisfied. Or even if you are eating what you want, maybe you are telling yourself that you really shouldn't be eating it, or are questioning or doubting your food choices.

Mindfulness and presence are powerful solutions. Awareness will not only help you tune in, listen to your body, and figure out what you really want and need, but it will also help you notice the textures, colors, smells, and flavors of your food. Eating is a sensory experience, after all, and one which we can enjoy when paying attention.

Making this shift—from fear and anxiety with our food, to more objectivity first and then positivity and peace—can improve your physical health while helping you to develop a better relationship with food. Furthermore, it may be the ticket to what you have been searching for all along if you have a history of dieting: peace with your food, body, and self.

As the *Course of Miracles* teaches, there is only ever fear and love.[26] When you up-level to love with your food, you will automatically feel more pleasure while eating. Although this might sound far-fetched at first, feeling pleasure positively impacts your metabolism and digestion. Remember, it isn't just about what you are eating—*how* you are eating matters, but the emotions you experience while you are eating play a role as well.

Taking biochemistry into consideration once again, there is a chemical released in your brain, specifically in your hypothalamus, that is associated with your pleasure response. Dopamine is produced when we eat the macronutrients protein and fat, and works to aid digestion, decrease appetite, and stimulate pleasure sensations in our cerebral cortex. We don't often think that pleasure has anything to do with appetite or metabolism, but it does, both from an emotional perspective and a biochemical one. With a lack of pleasure, your brain releases another chemical called neuropeptide Y; this amino acid neuropeptide is responsible for increasing appetite and tells us to search for food. It is naturally elevated in the morning and whenever we feel deprived of sustenance.[27] Studies have shown that it is also elevated when participants are on a restrictive diet, experiencing low blood sugar, and even in a low mood. When this is the case, neuropeptide Y makes us crave carbohydrates.[28]

We can assume then that if you are dieting, restricting, or otherwise denying yourself pleasure with the food you are eating, your body *will* demand it. It is a biological need and without it, your body will rebel. Again, this has nothing to do with your lack of "willpower" and everything to do with your brain, chemical makeup, and survival instincts.

What can you do to ensure more mindfulness, presence, and pleasure during your meals? Here are my favorite tips:

Breathe. Sometimes when I am eating in a public place, I notice others around me shoveling food in their mouths without coming up for air; this is detrimental, as our bodies need oxygen for optimal metabolism. Lining the interior of your small intestine, there are finger-like villi that are responsible for extracting the nutrients from your food. Given that your intestinal villi need oxygen from the blood to break-down and assimilate nutrients, when we don't slow down and breathe, oxygen decreases, which in turn decreases nutrient absorption. When nutrient absorption decreases, metabolism and fuel stores decrease (and energy suffers as well).

Now let's look at it from the perspective of the quality of your breath: Remember, if your breathing is shallow and quick, that could signal to your body that you are in a stressed-out sympathetic nervous state. But when your breathing is low, slow, and deep, that is characteristic of the calm, mindful parasympathetic state. Your breath alone is a tool you can use to dictate to your brain and body your state of being. Elongate your inhales and exhales while paying attention to the rhythm of your breathing, pause between bites, and supply your body with adequate oxygen.

Chew your food. Chewing is a mechanical action that is part of the eating process for a reason. Not only does it initiate the release of saliva, which contains essential enzymes to start breaking down your food, but it also helps to send the message to your brain that you are in fact eating. It locks in that mind-body connection. Additionally, this one act alone could help relieve any digestive distress and increase energy. Although you might not be able to feel it each time, digestion is a labor-intensive process. Your gut works *very* hard to do its job. The more you can break-down your food in your mouth before you even swallow, the less work your digestive tract must do, which can lead to an overall improved assimilation of nutrients; as a result, you might feel an increased sense of energy and satiation. I once heard an Ayurvedic practitioner say that for optimal digestion, our food should be the consistency of baby puree when we swallow. How many of you can say this is true for you? I will be honest, I would have to be very mindful—and chew *a lot*—in order for this to be true for me.

Eat without distractions. Put down your phone, close your computer, and turn off the television. Be there with your meal. Sit at a surface where you can create a beautiful space by setting the table, using a pretty plate, and lighting a candle; these small details make a difference. If you are not able to do this for every meal, try it once or twice.. This experimentation will give you a point of reference for comparison when you do eat in a more distracted state. How do you feel both physically and emotionally after eating mindfully versus distracted? You may now feel more motivated to create a more mindful experience with your meal even if you are multitasking. You still have the ability to pause, focus on your food, breathe, chew, and then go back to what you are doing.

Rethink portion control. So often, controlling portions is thought of in terms of the calories contained. Going forward, I want you to think about it differently from the perspective of energy and digestive efficiency. As I stated previously, digestion takes up a lot of energy and effort. When we eat to the point of feeling overly full (and then immediately feel tired), it is because you have put your gut into overload and it can't keep up. Think about eating to the point of lightness and energy as eating an amount where your stomach still has enough room to "churn," so to speak; otherwise, it can lead to issues such as heartburn and acid reflux. This mindset shift changes portion control from a place of denial or restriction to instead looking at it through the lens of self-care and ensuring your body has the ability to work efficiently. This principle not only applies to the amount you eat but to the speed in which you eat as well. Slowing down can help ensure you are eating to the point of energy and satiety, while supporting healthy digestion.

Express gratitude. Whether it is before you start eating or during your meal, pause and give thanks for the food on your plate (during this pause it might be a good time to take three deep breaths!). Gratitude and appreciation for the food in front of you will lead to a more pleasurable eating experience. Notice and savor the beauty of the food—the various colors that might be present on your plate—or put it into perspective by being thankful there is healthy food to eat. When pleasure is present, the body and mind will respond in a more positive way.

According to Jon Kabat-Zinn, meditation teacher, professor, and founder of MBSR (mindfulness-based stress reduction), the eating experience (and I would include the meal preparation leading up to eating) offers multiple moments each day to practice mindfulness. In his book *Wherever You Go, There You Are*, he asks, "Are you tasting your food? Are you aware of how fast, how much, when, where, and what you are eating? Can you make your entire day as it unfolds into an occasion to be present or to bring yourself back to the present, over and over again?"[29]

Mealtime can be an associative trigger to drop into the present moment; a reminder to be fully in the experience from which you flow (I will discuss flow in a later chapter). If formal meditation isn't something you are ready to tackle, eating is a good opportunity to start to observe the way your mind works. How is it trying to take you out of the present? With what thoughts? Where does your mind typically drift off to? Your family, job, or self-deprecating dialogue? Asking yourself these questions helps you pay attention to your attention.

Even after decades of doing mindfulness work himself, Kabat-Zinn describes his "humanness" of which we can all relate: "[The impulse to not be present] would have me eat breakfast with my eyes riveted to the cereal box, reading for the hundredth time…It scavenges to fill time, conspires with my mind to keep me unconscious, lulled in a fog of numbness to a certain extent, just enough to overfill my belly while I actually eat breakfast."

I will be the first to tell you that I constantly need to remember to eat more mindfully. As soon as I sit down, my hands want to open my laptop or pick up my phone; my mind wants to remind me of everything I have to do. The beautiful thing about the *practice* is that even if I drift, awareness disrupts it, and I am able to return to mindfulness. I feel the pull to distraction and bring myself back to the present. Some days are better than others, but I have made a deal with myself: If I choose to eat while doing other things, every time I take a bite, I am fully taking a bite. I am chewing my food. It is only after I have finished the bite that I can return to the activity. I compartmentalize, and this works for me.

The practice comes with the noticing; if your mind wanders off, bring it back. During meals, turn your attention back to your food—the taste, texture, and smells, what you are doing with your hands, and the colors at the end of your fork.

At the end of the book, you will find real food recipes to help you practice Counting Colors. Each one has been created with the philosophy in mind.

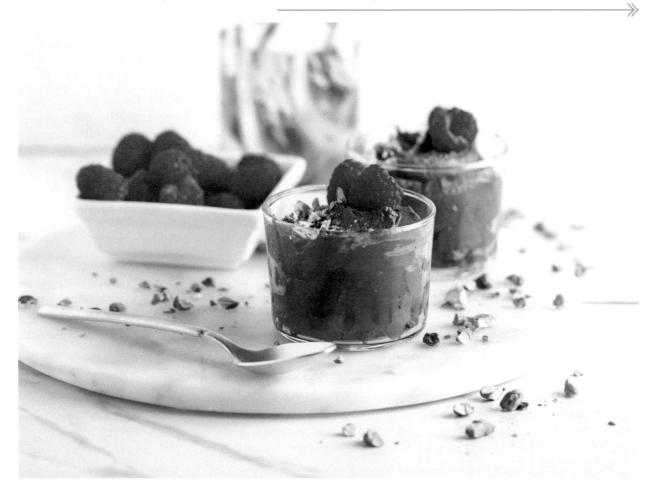

chapter five:
The Power of Your Thoughts

*W*hen I teach yoga, I like to weave in mantras and little messages on mindfulness. During one class in particular, I started to talk about the ego and thoughts, and how the noisy mental chatter that tends to rule our mindset is distinguishable from the essence of "you," or your intuition. After class, one of my students walked up to me hesitantly and asked, "Sara, what do you mean your thoughts are not you? Aren't the thoughts you think, that voice in your head, *you?*"

It can be a hard concept to grasp, but if you can observe and watch your thoughts, then they must be separate from your "self." Author Michael Singer in his bestselling book *The Untethered Soul* also makes this distinction: "If you're hearing [the voice inside your head] talk, it's obviously not you...you are the one who is aware of it...you are not the voice of the mind—you are the one who hears it."[30]

This isn't to say that your thoughts do not matter—they do. Your thoughts are powerful. Your inner dialogue and the way you speak both to yourself and about the situation at hand helps to create your reality, or your perception of reality at any given moment. I not only want you to realize the impact that they have on your relationship with food, your body, and your overall health, I eventually want you to consider the effects they are having in your daily life and your relationship with yourself.

Remember Brooke Castillo's model of thinking and emotions I mentioned earlier:

> *Your thoughts create your emotions; your emotions create your actions; your actions lead to results.*

If I was to ask you to analyze your inner dialogue around food, eating, exercise, and your body, how would you characterize them? Are they positive, nurturing, compassionate, or loving? Or are they the opposite? Do the words "should" and "shouldn't" often appear in your vocabulary? Do you beat yourself up, feel guilty or frustrated? And why is thinking about your thoughts in this way important?

Reflecting on your thoughts allows you to step out of a passive role and into an active one; it immediately means you become an observer. I am going to go into more detail about this when I discuss meditation and more abstract applications of this ability in your daily life, but keeping it in the realm of your physical health, your thoughts can affect you physiologically.

For example, your thoughts about a food are either going to have you feel a positive emotion or a negative one. It is then your emotional state that will impact your digestion, metabolism, and nutrient absorption.

There is a nerve that runs the length of your spinal cord from your brain all the way down to your digestive tract called the Vagus nerve, and it's the highway of communication between these two systems. Your mind is constantly communicating with your gut. It's a major reason why you can't separate the way you eat from the way you feel, not only physically but mentally as well, and why mental health issues, such as anxiety, depression, and attention deficit disorder (ADD), have been linked to inflammation in the gut.[31]

Let's paint a picture of when thoughts are positive before eating a certain food. I first learned about this phenomenon from Marc David's *The Slow Down Diet* and it has completely changed the way I eat. You are about to enjoy a slice of your birthday cake during a celebration with friends and family. You currently feel happy, calm, and peaceful. Not only are you surrounded by your loved ones but it's also your favorite kind of cake, so of course you are excited to enjoy it. In this situation, your hypothalamus (a small collection of tissues in the front part of your brain, which is responsible for integrating the activities of the mind with the biology of the body) will take this positive state of being and work to activate the parasympathetic nervous system response. Your body will turn on the "rest and digest" capabilities, and you will experience a more adequate breakdown of the calories (defined simply as the units of energy) in the cake, resulting in an increase in your body's ability to burn the calories (or energy) more efficiently.

Now let's consider a scenario on the opposite end of the spectrum. Due to years of dieting, restricting, and body image issues, you perceive eating a piece of cake as being "bad" and therefore something associated with feelings of guilt and shame (whether consciously or subconsciously). The thought of "I shouldn't be eating this sugar-filled food" floods your mind. Your body would then be sent into the sympathetic nervous state, impairing digestion, decreasing nutrient absorption, and slowing metabolism. Because peristalsis (gut motility) has slowed, the piece of cake may even stay in your digestive tract longer, creating constipation and harming the healthy bacteria. Your body is unable to efficiently break down and burn the energy it received from the cake. Furthermore, constipation and a build-up of waste in your digestive tract increases estrogen, which slows down your fat-burning capabilities. The only difference in these two scenarios: your emotional state before you ate.

What is important to remember is that every individual person is going to have different thoughts and emotions before each meal. Your thoughts around food and your relationship with food are very closely tied in to your "story" and long-held beliefs. Our past experiences are going to affect our present-day perceptions. I have seen this clearly exemplified with one of my best friends and me. She has always had a very positive relationship with food, while I—as you have learned from my story—have not. She has never been on a diet yet always stayed fit and trim; I battled my weight for over a decade. She never complained of stomach issues or food sensitivities, while I was at the mercy of mine for years. She would always stop when satisfied and never really thought about food between meals; food was always on my mind, and I would eat as if it was my last meal every time.

Fortunately, we are not at the mercy of this story, and we have the ability to rewrite it.

journal:

Earlier, I wanted you to reflect and journal on your health journey thus far; now I want you to reflect on your relationship with food. How would you describe it currently and how would you like it to be different? As you write, try not to judge yourself for the type of relationship you have had up until this point. There is no good or bad, there is no right or wrong, and there is no normal—there just is. Notice, acknowledge, and, if you would like to take it a step further, envision how you want to feel.

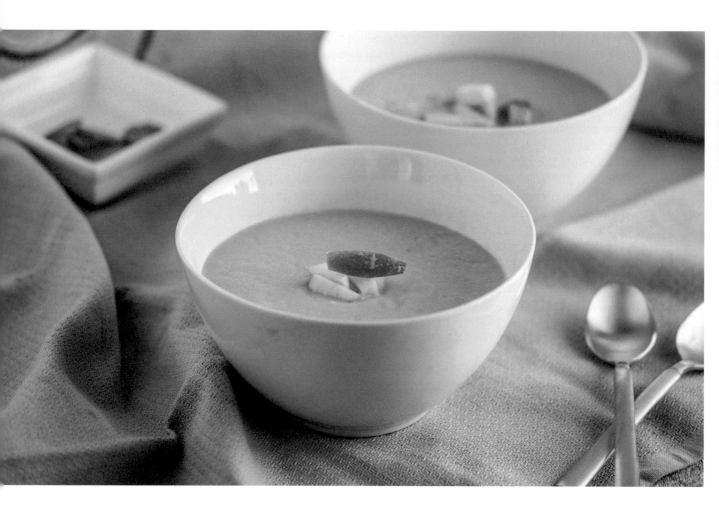

chapter six:

PRACTICING THE ART OF NON-JUDGMENT

*I*n almost every initial health consultation I conduct with my clients, I hear judgment around the way one eats, categorizing food as "good" or "bad." *I was eating so well for a while and then fell off the wagon; during the work week I am being "good" with my food and exercise, and then the weekend rolls around and my healthy habits go to hell in a hand basket.* Does this sound familiar? I know I can relate.

Essentially, when you speak this way, whether you realize it or not, you are attaching your morality to the food you eat or the exercise you did or did not do. In return, even if it is on a subconscious level, you are doing your emotional well-being a huge disservice, as you then may feel negative emotions, such as guilt and shame, as a result.

There is no such thing as "good' or "bad" food—it is neutral. Food is what it is made of; it is the nutrients it provides (or doesn't provide); it is the textures, colors, and smells. Right away when you put something into a camp of good versus bad, you are judging and labeling something that is not inherently moral, and from *this* arises the emotions attached to the judgment.

As a human, know that this is completely natural. Our brains are very efficient, so these labels serve a purpose: they are meant to provide mental shortcuts so we don't have to think so hard, and they are completely tied to our past experiences with whatever it is we are labeling. It helps our brains conserve energy, make quick decisions, and take action. This is a survival instinct, and because it is the way of your mind or ego, it is essentially rooted in fear. It is meant to keep you alive. Yet these judgments and thoughts are not reality. What is real has no judgment; reality is always neutral. Increasing consciousness and awareness is the only antidote, as intellectually, our minds cannot fully grasp this concept.

When it comes to food specifically, I encourage you to change your language by making it more objective. While there might not be good and bad food, there is *nutritious* and *non-nutritious*; there are those foods that serve you and those that do not. These foods are going to be different for *everyone*, which is why blanket approaches to nutrition do not work, and why you cannot base the way you eat off of someone else and what they are doing.

Take almonds for example. The reality of the situation is that, objectively, almonds are a tree nut and contain nutrition, specifically protein, fiber, antioxidants, vitamins like vitamin E and riboflavin, and minerals such as magnesium and calcium. If I was to tell someone this, they would likely say almonds are a nutritious food. But what if you have a tree nut allergy? If you eat an almond, you go into anaphylactic shock. Almonds are literally your poison, so to you, they are quite the opposite. They are a very non-nutritious food and do not serve your physical health.

This is the magic of tuning in to your body, what it needs and wants, asking the right questions, and responding in an informed way. Be curious and release any need for perfection—it doesn't exist. There also are no absolutes.

There are those less-nutritious foods we eat due to taste and experience that might not serve a nutritional purpose, but they bring us joy in the moment, and that is what life is about: creating experiences that make us feel joy. I call these foods *soul-nourishing* versus cell-nourishing. If choosing to eat a less-nutritious food results in stress, anxiety, and guilt, then I advise you to either view the experience through a more positive lens (which you have complete control over), or to choose a more nutritious choice instead. Every one of these situations is going to look different, which is what moment-to-moment awareness is all about. Sometimes you will eat the cake, and sometimes you know it might not serve you in that moment, so you choose not to. This is what being more present with your choices is all about. Realizing that you have this choice in the first place is true empowerment.

A mental tip I like to offer in these types of experiences is what I call "playing the whole tape," which can help bring a new level of awareness to your decision making. A therapist once taught this theory to me; it had nothing to do with food but pertained to another area of my life in which I was making poor choices. After hearing it, a big light bulb went off that forever changed my thinking. As humans, we are creatures of instant gratification. We love the quick fix, and the faster we can feel good, the better. Societal marketing and advertising is centered around this phenomenon.

When you incorporate the concept of playing the whole tape, however, you consider the long-term effects of your behavior *in the moment* in order to avoid any negative residual ramifications. This is one brain "power" we humans have over other animals: We can visualize how a present moment circumstance could affect us in the future. Playing the whole tape also takes consciousness, because subconscious programming is strong, and breaking the habit of making decisions to reap immediate rewards could take some work. You have to use awareness to pause before making a decision in order to play the tape in the first place.

Dr. John Sarno, author of the bestselling book *The Mindbody Prescription*, argues that "although most people think decision making is the domain of the conscious mind, actually it is a process that draws upon all that has been learned and felt in the past, including information that resides in the unconscious."[32] Therefore, to create change and feel more empowered in your choices and behavior, it is about bringing the preprogramming to the surface through awareness, getting real with the deeply rooted ruts in which you have been riding along until now, understanding what has been habit or tied to limiting beliefs, and taking the baby action steps you need to take to step more fully into a healthier, happier version of you.

When it comes to your food choices, you can play the whole tape by asking how the food will make you *feel* a little bit later than the first five minutes. Often, this means forgoing the instant gratification of a less-nutritious choice in order to eat in a way that better serves you. Remember, the brain, body, and ego love instant satisfaction, and if stubborn, your mind is going to want what it wants, when it wants it, and usually that means immediately. A simple visualization exercise can be helpful. You may have to call on past experiences for information to support your decision-making process. Whether it is with an individual meal, a social event, or an entire weekend, envision how you want to feel both during and after. Put pen to paper if you have to. Then take the small action steps and choose the foods and beneficial behaviors that will get you there. The same can be said for other types of choices as well.

I want to clarify that when it comes to tuning in, making choices, and even playing the whole tape, that you are always doing so from a place of allowance and permission. You are never telling yourself that you can't or shouldn't have something; I want you to do the opposite—I want you tell yourself that you can eat anything you want (yes, anything!). Give yourself that permission. We human beings are a funny bunch. You tell us we can't have something, and we are going to want it even more. Tell us not to push the big red button or think of a purple elephant, and, well, you know what happens. Whether it was a toy when you were young, a boy in college, or a chocolate truffle at a cocktail party, according to biochemistry, if we are told it is unattainable, it is going to be mighty difficult to fight that desire. If this wiring lives on a subconscious level, your behavior will be more automatic, and you will find yourself choosing something even when you *know* it isn't good for you.

For example, I love a good glass of wine and decadent cheese plate. Over the years when we have gone out to eat, my husband and I have ordered the delicious duo to begin our meal. I am aware now that there was a strong association with eating in a restaurant and splurging on this appetizer. It had become a special occasion, so how could I say no? It was the rebel in me coming out to play. Some of you may be rolling your eyes at the idea of being rebellious over some fine cheese and fig jam, but I *knew* at the time (and still know) I am intolerant to some dairy, so health-wise, it wasn't in my best interest to order it. Every time I ate it, I paid the price. I would wake up in the middle of the night with stomach cramps, or my face would break out the next day. My body felt inflamed. I started to take a taste of my own medicine. If I saw a cheese plate on the appetizer menu, I would give myself permission; I would tell myself I could order it. But did I want to? Then I would play the whole tape to the sleepless night and stomachache. It was only then that I developed the clarity and willpower to pass on it with ease.

Part of this "want what we can't have" occurrence has to do with curiosity. The Information-Gap Theory was developed by George Lowenstein, economics and psychology professor at Carnegie Mellon University. In his research paper titled *The Psychology of Curiosity*, he states that "Curiosity has consistently been recognized as a critical motive that influences human behavior in both positive and negative ways...[and] poses an anomaly for rational-choice analysis of behavior."[33] When you are told you can't have something, your subconscious mind immediately starts to question and wonder why. Rational thinking is clouded by rebellion. Before you know it, your behavior is being controlled by your brain's need to quench the curiosity. Your decision making is strongly influenced by this subconscious programming, even if you know a certain choice does not serve your greater good.

As if that isn't enough, brain chemistry plays a role as well. When we want something, the mere thought of the desire triggers our reward hormone dopamine to rise—and continue to rise the longer we wait for it.[34] The more you are denied (or deny yourself) the object of your affection, the stronger the desire grows. This is another reason why dieting, denial, and restriction around what you truly want will likely backfire. These survival reactions and responses are not easy to fight. After years of having rules around food, this might seem scary to some of you to give yourself that permission, worried that if you are not holding yourself to familiar standards to keep yourself "safe," you will eat anything and everything. That could be the case, and the fear will feel more real only if you don't trust yourself. Self-trust is so important. This is another mindset shift if it is something that is unfamiliar for you, and can be the most challenging, but it is a game-changer.

You and your body were built to be a team. The goals and values of both are the same: for *you* to navigate, survive, and thrive through life. Know that the "you" I am referring to can't be reduced to just your mind or your body, which I will talk more about when we get more into the spirituality side of things. Unfortunately, over time this bond can get broken. Maybe some health issues happened, and you felt like your body failed you; perhaps you don't feel good and energized in your body, so the negative self-talk has created a chasm that keeps on getting wider every time you look in the mirror. If one thing breaks the bond between you and your body, it's the self-deprecating record that continuously plays in your mind.

Another big trust breaker is the cycle I often see with my clients: the yo-yo dieting, the ups and downs, the restriction, over-consumption, over-exercising, more restriction, and around it goes. Your body thrives on predictability; it needs to trust that it will be nourished. Without this trust, it basically lives in survival mode and is consistently stressed out, staying in that sympathetic nervous system state; remember, that state of being doesn't do your physical or emotional health any favors. What I want to reiterate is that your body needs to trust that it will be *nourished*, not simply fed. You have likely heard the saying used to define our society: over-fed and under-nourished. The whole, real foods with the one ingredient information are what your body needs to thrive.

Make the commitment to trust yourself; trust that you will use your intuition to make mindful food choices for you and your body. Tune in, listen, honor your cravings, and make the most informed choice. This is teamwork! Your body will tell you both what and how much it needs. Along these lines, trust that you will stop when satisfied. And lastly, trust that you will allow yourself to indulge every once in a while without overdoing it. Practice the mindset of peace and permission. Your body is your best compass. It will tell you what and how much it needs, and the more you make that mind-body connection, the stronger your bond becomes. Especially important, speak kindly to your body, fuel it with high-vibrational foods, show yourself compassion and love, and build that beautiful relationship. Let go of the need to over-control and really trust yourself. This is true empowerment over your health.

In her book *A Return to Love*, Marianne Williamson illustrates this shift so beautifully:

> When I was in my twenties, I had a problem with weight—not enough of a problem to be called fat, but enough to keep me miserable. There was a problematic ten to fifteen pounds that I could never shake. Anytime I went on a diet, I ended up gaining weight. This makes sense psychologically, because if someone tells us not to think about the Eiffel Tower, we will think about it all the time. Telling myself not to think about food only made me more obsessed about it. Deprivation is a lousy way to lose weight. I used to pray about my problem and would receive the following guidance: "Eat anything you want." That sounded thoroughly insane to me. "But if I tell myself to do that," I thought, "then I'll start eating and I'll never stop." To that my internal guidance responded, "Yes, you will do that at first. You will have to compensate for all of the pressure you've been putting on yourself for years. And then you will have had enough. Then you will return to your natural rhythms. Then you will heal."

> So I let go. I decided that it didn't matter how much I weighed. I couldn't take the horror of the obsession anymore. What I realized was that my weight had nothing to do with my body, but with my mind. My ego's purpose for the weight was to keep me separate, and until I gave up that purpose, I would never be able to give up the extra pounds. My subconscious mind was merely following instructions.

> [What I learned was that] the point of healthy food is that it supports us in existing the most lightly and energetically within the body. It is the heavier, unhealthy food that ties us to the body. We take care of the body as a way of taking better care of the spirit.[35]

What her story encompasses is one of the greatest mindset shifts of all: the one to self-love.

To make sustainable changes, whether it is with your food choices, behavior, or those habits that are not serving you, it will be a lot more motivating to make these changes when you approach them from a place of self-love and respect rather than restriction and fear. For example, with your food: choosing to eat whole, real foods instead of processed foods because you know they *benefit* you, and you love and respect your body (and self) enough to nourish it with nutrients. When you shift your perspective to become more positive about both food and your body, you start to view food in this way, not as something to make you feel guilty, ashamed, or anxious. If you have yet to love yourself, this is where the deeper inner work needs to occur, because remember: If you don't like something deep down, you aren't really going to care about how you treat it. The restriction mentality often stems from a *fear* of something, whether that is gaining weight or otherwise, which is also wrapped in a lack of self-trust or self-love. Restriction serves a purpose of punishment, control, assuaging guilt, or reinforcing subconscious negative beliefs.

According to psychiatrist and international bestselling author Elisabeth Kübler-Ross, there only ever is fear and love.[36] Most of us are walking around in a cloudy fog of the former. There is a disconnect between the intuitive love we are born with and the way we feel about ourselves on the surface. The more you bring consciousness to your intuition and innate sense of love, the more you will discover and uncover what is true for you.

In his book *The Slow Down Diet*, Marc David categorizes love as one of the "eight sacred metabolizers." In other words, feelings that not only create a positive environment in the body, but bring us closer to a higher power:

By embodying [the eight sacred metabolizers] we become more like the source from whence we came, more of who we are meant to be and who we know somewhere inside, we want to be. [They] have been classically viewed as qualities or traits, not material quantities unto themselves. And yet I would say that every sacred metabolizer is both a force and a substance...Somewhere in the body, love molecules squirt about when feelings of love are activated...First comes the thought or feeling, then comes the molecule.[37]

According to David, the other seven sacred metabolizers are truth, courage, commitment, compassion, forgiveness, faith, and surrender. With regards to faith, it is important to clarify that you can't simply tell yourself you love yourself; you must feel it—you must *believe* it. The power of belief (which I will talk more about) and the subconscious mind play a fundamental role in your reality and behavior.

In his book *The Biology of Belief*, Bruce Lipton states that "the mere thinking of positive thoughts will not necessarily have any impact on our lives at all" due to the difference of the conscious mind and subconscious programming.[38] The conscious mind is where we hold our desires; it is also where we can call upon positive thinking. The subconscious, however, is not only stronger than surface-level thinking but habitual and basically in the driver's seat of our actions. Many of our beliefs and behaviors are stored in our subconscious, which rules approximately 95% of our experience. It controls a lot of the habits of our physical body. It is what explains your ability to drive a car from point A to point B without really remembering the ride.

What is important to realize is that your subconscious was shaped at a very early age, typically by age eight. As you read in my story, a comment made about my body in childhood planted a seed of belief that caused me to feel shame; reciting a positive affirmation that "my body is beautiful" contradicts this early established belief. It took deeper work to deprogram and rewire new beliefs. If this resonates with you, it could also require digging a bit deeper, unblocking those deep-seated beliefs or whatever it is that is holding you back from stepping into the highest and most loving version of yourself.

Any negativity, self-deprecation, or victimization are all ways your ego keeps you "safe" by keeping you scared. Yet these negative thoughts are not what is real. We are all energetic beings of love. It takes practice, and if you were to get very quiet, be in the present moment, and clear the noise and mental chatter, you would feel more peaceful. You would be able to tap into a more loving place, and what is hopeful is that we all have the ability to get there. It is a practice because this work is not about perfection; that doesn't exist, so give yourself permission to let perfectionistic tendencies go. As a human being, you will make mistakes. You may even make decisions that do not serve you. Your mind will wander to negative spaces both in meditation and in daily life; this is the natural tendency of the mind and will always be the case as long as you are alive. Beating yourself up will only make things worse. Self-love is about showing *compassion* for ourselves despite the "humanness."

Self-love was always the missing piece to my emotional eating puzzle. The way I felt about myself on the inside had everything to do with my tendency to binge and restrict. To clarify, emotional eating can take many different forms. Even if you are not someone who has binged, if you have had instances when you felt a negative emotion—loneliness, sadness, boredom, anger, frustration, stress—and eaten food in response to that emotion when you were not *physically* hungry, I would characterize that as emotional eating.

Since negative emotions alone can instigate a stress response, it is highly related to eating habits: cortisol increases, blood sugar spikes and then subsequently drops, and because your body is going to want to get back into balance (homeostasis), you will likely crave the foods that are going to bring blood sugar back up quickly (i.e. carbohydrates and sugar), and the cycle continues. Compound that with the fact that these foods produce the happy chemicals in your brain, and again, you have a strong conditioning that is hard to break.

Author, teacher, and emotional-eating expert Geneen Roth states that when working through negative emotions, food can't do that for you.[39] To use food to numb or soothe does not do the trick, even if it feels that way immediately. It is highly likely that whichever negative emotion you are feeling (such as sadness, boredom, loneliness) will eventually be replaced by another (guilt, shame, anger). I also want to make it clear that I am not saying emotional eating is "bad" or wrong in any way. If you have ever felt the effects of emotional eating, you might feel powerless, a lack of control, or on autopilot in the face of it. The more this cycle occurs, the more we are conditioned to seek out the behavior. Because in the short-term, it seems to be very effective.

To illustrate the emotional eating cycle:

Having a negative thought leads to having a negative emotion. The negative emotion is uncomfortable, so one tries to find a way out of the discomfort. In the case of emotional eating, it's food (other examples of numbing mechanisms include alcohol, shopping, sex). Because our minds love instant gratification, we turn to those foods that make us feel happy and bring comfort and relief in the short-term, not considering (i.e. playing the whole tape) how they might make us feel a little later. The behavior creates a (false) sense of immediate gratification, and your brain remembers that; it creates a mental shortcut so when you feel a similar negative emotion in the future, your mind will tell you to engage in the same behavior as a response. Again, this conditioning can be very strong, which might be why you feel powerless. It might even be something you are telling yourself over and over: *I feel powerless in the face of food. I am not in control.* Because you keep telling yourself this, whether consciously or subconsciously, that is what you believe. What you believe plays such a large role in creating your reality. According to the Law of Attraction, you could be manifesting experiences that reinforce those beliefs.

In hindsight, I see this in my story—you may see it in yours. It repeatedly occurred when I was caught in my cycle. Most of my binge eating happened after I had consumed too much alcohol, and I believe that when I was in that state, something was triggered in my brain to associate binge eating with feeling better. Then consider the fact that if you drink alcohol, blood sugar spikes and then drops very quickly, and your body craves those carb-heavy foods in order to bring your blood sugar back up. For me to break this cycle of behavior (aside from taking a long break from drinking alcohol), I had to get to the root of the issue; I had to directly face the fact that I was self-medicating for the uncomfortable emotions I was feeling.

My antidote was both mindfulness and self-empowerment. Educating myself on everything I have talked about to this point also played a role in my healing. I had to realize I was not powerless, I was in control, and so are you. If we have control over one thing in this life, it's our thoughts and how we respond to our thoughts, situations, and circumstances. It might not feel that way sometimes, but it's true. The solution isn't in analyzing and trying to change the surface-level behavior (the emotional eating, for instance), it is analyzing and getting real with your thoughts and emotional frequency. I say "frequency" because I want you to think about your emotions on a scale. We have the ability to turn the dial in order to achieve a higher-frequency emotion.

If you are someone who is intimidated by meditation (which I will discuss later) or not yet ready to adopt a formal practice, there is a simple exercise you can do to bring more awareness to your thoughts and emotions; I call it the "Do You Sing in the Shower Exercise." What better place to become an objective observer of your thoughts?

Do You Sing in the Shower?

I believe the shower to be the prime time to analyze your emotional frequency. To sing in the shower may sound more like a cliché than something people actually do, but there are people out there who do in fact sing in the shower.

When I think about taking a shower, most of the time I'm going through the motions and my mind is a million miles away. My thoughts are running through my list of to-dos, or replaying a situation in the past and how I could have gone about it differently, or creating future scenarios and how I will handle them, even if they haven't happened yet, and even if they probably won't happen. It's exhausting, and half the time I ask myself whether or not I just shampooed my hair. I step out with more anxiety than when I walked in, with that familiar hurried feeling to get to the next thing. Rarely do I notice the color, shape, and feel of the shampoo bottle or lather of the suds or the sensation of running water on my skin.

If you shower once a day, this gives you a daily opportunity to *practice* noticing. Noticing your thoughts, where your mind wanders, and observe what comes up for you. What I want you to eventually realize is that mindfulness isn't about trying to control your thoughts and emotions; that's not the point. Your mind will wander—it's inevitable. It's about continuing to catch yourself in those moments, and then gently and with compassion, bringing your mind back to the present. Another reason why the shower is a great time to practice awareness is because, similar to eating, it is a sensory experience and one in which your hands are doing something the entire time (washing your hair, lathering your loofa, shaving your legs). I have heard creatives say the shower is a prime time for dreaming up future projects. Not only is it a good time to witness your individual frequency, but there is also something about being intentionally present in the shower that is conducive for idea generation. In fact, the tagline for this book came to me in the shower. I can tell you that likely would not have happened if I was worried about an upcoming conference call or what I was going to fix for dinner.

Know that you can tune in to your frequency and practice presence at any time. My life coach Ellie Burke once taught me that our hands have a lot of energy. The physical sensations of the body in a given moment are great tools to help you feel present (one of the many benefits of yoga), but by paying attention to your hands especially—which seem to always be in the act of something—it serves to snap you back into awareness. Whether you are preparing your food or actually eating, your hands are engaged. Remember this mnemonic the next time you are making your meal, but also know you can bring it off your plate and apply it to your daily life: notice your hands on the steering wheel while driving to work; brushing your child's hair in the morning; sifting through the mail in the evening.

As I dive deeper into emotional frequency in a later chapter, you will learn that your emotions can be viewed as information, just as I described your cravings are information. In his book *You Are the Placebo*, New York Times bestselling author Dr. Joe Dispenza says just as "thoughts are the language of the brain, emotions are the language of the body."[40] Emotions can be viewed as internal signals that something occurring either in your external world or with your thoughts is either aligning or misaligning with your sense of inner peace, or your intuition. By becoming an observer and then engaging in a self-guided inquiry process, you can empower yourself to change your inner environment. You will also learn that to "turn up the dial" on your emotional frequency, you can't just close your eyes and will yourself to a more positive emotion. You must peel back the layers of your thoughts and release the ego's need to be right or stay "safe." It takes work to change your thoughts and mental habituations of the mind.

Avoid feeling like you need to control your thoughts or completely clear your mind. The practice is more about that moment of consciousness; the "waking up" and realizing that your thoughts are in the past or in the future, after which you gently guide your awareness back to the sensory experience in front of you and the way you feel in your body. Each moment is only ever a neutral experience. Our minds filter the moment, attaching labels and judgments, which then turn it into either a negative or positive one. I went over this as it pertains to your food, but it can be the case for anything. This is how our story and lens through which we look at life influence our present reality, even when the past and projected future have nothing to do with it.

When it comes to your emotional frequency, you can think of this as your mood or baseline state of being. Your emotions will be influenced by your thoughts at any given moment. Maybe you describe the thoughts in your mind as chaotic, constantly running every waking hour. According to research conducted by the National Science Foundation, a person on average has 12,000 to 60,000 thoughts per day. Of those thoughts, 80 percent are negative. What is more, 95 percent of those negative thoughts are repetitive.[41] Think about that: The human mind is basically a broken record of pessimism. No wonder we can be our own worst critics or go through life holding a half-empty glass. It's simply part of the human condition for survival.

Your thoughts are going to be influenced by your perception, which is tied to your story, subconscious, childhood, and core beliefs; in other words, the programming from your past. Fortunately, none of this is set in stone. While neuroscientists once believed our brains were set at adolescence, we now know this is not the case. Evidence has established that the brain is "plastic," implying it can be rewired well into adulthood.[42] Not only is this empowering to know, but consciousness for the mental tendencies of your individual mind can also help break your conditioning. You may have thought and perceived this way for years, but it is not something you have to sustain. In any given moment, you have the opportunity to rewrite your story.

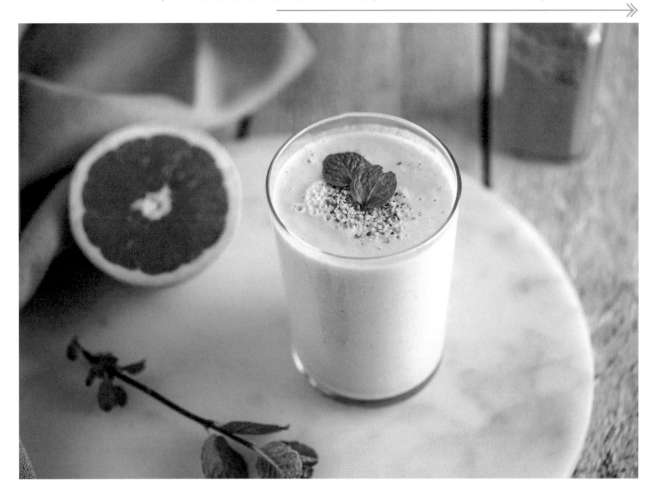

chapter seven:

REWRITE YOUR HEALTH STORY

i would argue that everyone has a vision for either better health or happiness. If you are someone who feels that you have already attained your physical goals, that is amazing! Perhaps you have a vision for an improved version of you: the "you" that is more aligned with the "you" you know you can be—this is natural. As humans, we have an innate desire to evolve, grow, and expand. If you have a vision for better health, trust that you can get there. In my health coaching practice, I help guide my clients toward their vision. If you are currently in a state you do not want to stay in (whether physically, mentally, emotionally), the first step is realizing that the way things have been is not the way things will always have to be.

Your intuition or your gut might be telling you there is more—something else you can be doing to be healthier, happier, and more whole. This does not make you a malcontent; we are supposed to *want* to become better and more aligned. This is your inner being craving wholeness. And know this: When it comes to achieving a more aligned state of being, it has little to do with your behavior. It isn't all about better nutrition and balance. It isn't about how much time you spend in the gym, how much sleep you get, or how much water you drink. It isn't about being perfect, and it isn't even about your physical body at all. Don't get me wrong—taking care of your physical body is a pathway to taking care of your energy, and even supporting better health and happiness, but it is more about the way you feel emotionally and the way your spirit feels *in* your body. That is where you need to bring your attention and focus after you have worked on the fundamentals I have discussed up to this point.

This is where your mindset and emotional frequency come into play—the thoughts running through your mind, the way you speak to yourself on a daily basis, and the beliefs you have that are influencing your thoughts, actions, and eventually results. If I have a client come to me who is struggling with low energy and fatigue, yet she feels as if she is eating a nutrient-dense diet, exercising, getting good sleep, and staying hydrated, I want to know how she is speaking to herself. I want to know where the imbalances are in the more abstract areas of her life: relationships, career, spirituality, and joy. It is not the first thing we think of, but voids in these areas are major energy drains.

Sometimes energy has nothing to do with the physical. Think about it: Have you ever had a time in your life when suddenly you had a rush of energy because your emotional state changed? Maybe you fell in love, received good news, or landed your dream job. The vibrancy and extra pep in your step did not stem from a change in your physical state but rather a change in your internal perception. The opposite can be true as well. Can you remember a time when you felt sad or even depressed, leaving you with a lack of energy and motivation?

In his book *The Untethered Soul*, Michael Singer proclaims we all have a wellspring of energy within that we can draw upon at any time, yet most of us block it. We block it with our thoughts, and we block it with our fear.[43] But when you open your awareness and you shift from fear to love, that's where the magic happens.

As long as we are alive, we are thinking beings; that is never going to change. We have a mind and we have an ego, and the ego is always going to tempt you to be in a place that is safe, familiar, and "comfortable." Remember, your mind is always going to try and preserve energy by creating shortcuts, telling you things like, "When this happened in the past, this occurred as a result, so if something similar is happening now, that must mean this..." If this thought pattern is creating self-limiting beliefs, then it is simply fear disguised as comfort. What is "comfortable" could be rooted in fear and creating that block. Unblocking is about increasing your awareness and attention for how you operate; for how your thoughts, perceptions, and beliefs are limiting you, ultimately making a shift from fear to love.

Psychiatrist Phil Stutz and psychotherapist Barry Michels, bestselling authors of *The Tools*, describe the comfort zone as a safe place to which we retreat to avoid discomfort and pain. For most people, it is not a physical place but rather a way of life—a deeply ingrained habit—to avoid anything that might cause us pain.[44]

The tendency to remain in your comfort zone is likely influenced by your past, or your "story." Often, your present is influenced by your past, which is why I want you to really reflect on your story. Your story *is* a part of you, and there is nothing you can do to change how everything unfolded up until this point; there is no need to try to change it or judge it, attaching those labels of right or wrong. Let it be, and then let it go. Use it as information without allowing it to tether you to a certain way of being.

There is a difference between allowing the past to negatively impact your present and using it as information. It is important not to cling to the past or allow past circumstances, events, behaviors, and beliefs to dictate your present if you don't want them to; however, you can use your past as information. Easier said than done, but it entails viewing your past with more of an objective lens. Circumstances can be looked upon as a lesson or an opportunity. The wonderful thing about being a free-thinking human is that you have the complete ability to make a change if that is what you want. Every *new* choice provides you the opportunity to make a change and align with your higher vision of self, whether it is in the action you take or the thoughts you think, and it starts with awareness to the potential of the present moment.

As a human, this can be difficult, given your self-constructed identity. The ego enjoys behavior that aligns with your sense of self, and anything that goes against what is familiar leads to discomfort. For example, if you weren't raised to value nutrition, and eating healthy food has not been an aspect of your experience (i.e. your "story"), and then you set a goal to eat healthier, the behavior might not be as sustainable if you attempt to achieve this goal under the preconceived notion of who you have always been. Every time you eat a salad or drink a green smoothie, there might be thoughts running in the background sounding a lot like, "What are you doing? This isn't who you are. You don't actually *like* healthy food!" Then bring in the underlying (and more complex) emotional layers of food relationships, and it is less about the goal to eat healthier, and more about the mindsets behind the goal. But if you flip the script and embrace the mindset of "someone who values eating healthy food," if you become someone who simply does what you want to do, you are much more likely to be successful. Each moment offers you the ability to choose who you are and align your behavior accordingly. Acknowledging and unblocking long-held beliefs about your "self" is the first step to creating desired change.

According to James Clear, author of *Atomic Habits*, "progress requires unlearning. Becoming the best version of yourself requires you to continuously edit your beliefs, and to upgrade and expand your identity."[45] To be fully absorbed in the present moment is the epitome of self-expansion. The possibilities are endless. You are neither limited nor influenced by the stories of your past or worries of your future. You *are* with the power to be.

The other side of this coin is to not project too much into the future; not to allow thoughts of sustaining that change five days, five months, or five years down the road paralyze you into inaction. The future hasn't happened yet—none of that is real. I want you to send all your energy to the present moment to tune in to *you*. Do what feels good and aligned in that moment, and unfold from there. I will expand more on this when I discuss the power of flow.

In our society, people tend to lose the connection to themselves and the present moment. It is why we are always looking to external sources for information, validation, and structure. People pay more attention to what this person is doing on Instagram, or what this expert is saying about what is right and good, and less attention to what is going on right in from of them and in their individual body. I frequently witness this in my health coaching practice.

For example, someone comes to me to lose weight. They want structure. They want to be told what to eat, when to eat, and how much to eat. They want easy. They want shortcuts, meal plans, and rules. The need for hand-holding is how we were raised, with teachers, parents, and coaches telling us what to do, how to be, and how to act. Furthermore, the ego loves easy and instant gratification. But I can't tell someone how to eat. I'm not in their body on any given day. I don't know the state of their hormones, the quality of their sleep, or the level of their activity. As a health coach, it is my responsibility to provide information and education, point to what the research says from an objective standpoint, guide someone to turn inward and pay attention to her internal signals, and help her practice making the mind-body connection and finding an inner alignment toward a good feeling place. That guidance—that teamwork—is what will set someone up for sustainable success.

Julie* (all names have been changed) came to me not only for weight loss and nutrition but also to really learn and understand the *why* behind her food choices. This desire is always a good start; intention coupled with understanding creates more motivation and increases the likelihood of staying on track.

In our initial consultation, she painted a picture of a history of dieting and depriving. Always having looked outside herself for answers and structure, it seemed as if she partook in a plan no matter what it was, as long as she had someone or something else telling her what to do. What was clearly missing in this approach was the foundational understanding of why she "should be" eating a certain way. Without this crucial component, she didn't stay motivated for long, and would then move on to the next plan or program. She finally met her breaking point when her last nutritionist, in response to her complaints about hunger and cravings, prescribed her a pill to help those "symptoms" subside. The medication made her moody and depressed, and she quickly stopped taking it (and subsequently fired her nutritionist).

Right before she reached out to me, she and her husband had just undergone a move to a new city, and she was entering a period when life was feeling a bit more settled, therefore wanting to focus on herself and physical health. While she revealed she no longer worked out or belonged to a gym, she was wanting to get back into exercise, yet she felt lost in terms of what to do.

Ironically, despite having disclosed that she was "not good" with diets, and instead wanting slow, steady, and sustainable change, she constantly requested more structure from me with her meals. Old mental habits die hard in this regard, and my answer was always the same: "In terms of when to eat and how much to eat, I can't tell you that. Your body is your best compass. My responsibility is to provide you the nutritional science and information behind real foods, a blood sugar balancing way of eating, but when it comes to the specific choices around your eating, only you can decide." The problem? Like so many of my clients, a lack of self-trust prevented Julie from fully embracing this belief. Yet for healthy habits to become a lifestyle, she had to be able to use the tools, information, and inner wisdom to guide her choices when her hand was no longer being held.

In our next few sessions together, we simultaneously spent the time talking about the nutritional science behind weight loss and food as information, and the mindset shifts that needed to occur around food and her relationship to it. It was my hope that through objective education, she would begin to develop her trust muscle around mealtime; in other words, that she had everything she needed to approach her health journey in a more positive way. Very early on I informed her of my Counting Colors philosophy: that every time she sat down to a meal, she should ask, *how is this food benefitting me? How is it serving the purpose of providing my body with nutrients?* Nutrients in our food are represented by an array of colors, from the bright orange of beta carotene, to the deep hue of blues and purples of anthocyanin, each affecting our physical body on a cellular level. Two main phenomena in our society prevent us from viewing food this way: the dieting culture and the Standard American Diet. Julie specifically had fallen susceptible to the former. Like so many women who have lived through the 1980s and 1990s, she held on to a more "black and white" belief: that all calories are created equal, and it didn't really matter where they came from as long as they fell under a certain number. Her work was not only to debunk that belief but to also change her language and release old ways of thinking that were standing in the way of her ideal vision of health.

In terms of her language around food, there existed a lot of judgment. Labeling food as "good" versus "bad," while also judging herself on what she wanted to be eating against what she felt like she "should" be eating. Over the next few months, I encouraged Julie to figure out what was true for her in any given moment, to become more present with her food and exercise, and to let go of the over-thinking. Essentially, I wanted her to ground herself in her physical body and flow from there. So often when it comes to our wellness, we reside in our minds, but that is quite backward. The majority of our wellness practices—from eating, to movement, to meditation—are to be *felt* in our physical body on a moment-to-moment basis.

What is interesting, and something I have witnessed many times before (even with myself), is that halfway through her health coaching program with me, she and her husband took a vacation. Upon her return, she explained how wonderful it was to stop obsessing and worrying; to let go of the rules and restrictions around her eating and exercise. In fact, she told me she gave herself permission to eat and enjoy, to not exercise, aside from oceanside strolls along the beach, and to relax and just *be*. Additionally, a separate struggle she had been facing was that having moved to a new city, she felt as if she wasn't contributing financially to her household. She had spent decades raising her children, and as newly empty nesters, she didn't have a job or "structure" to her day (do you see the parallel?). After having a candid conversation with her husband, he told her it was fine she didn't work, and encouraged her to start doing things outside the house that made her happy; with this, she felt a huge sense of relief. The result? She came home feeling lighter and more energized, the two feelings she had been searching for all along.

The dieting mentality and reliance on a plan or program with strict rules or restrictions cannot only cause you to lose that connection but also lose sight of what really matters: how you want to *feel* after achieving your goals. What are the emotions you are hoping to feel? Know that there is a difference between external goals and your internal intentions. Your internal intentions are the emotions. Staying with the weight-loss analogy, many want to lose weight not because it is about the number but because of how they feel once they achieve it; they think they will feel happier, more confident, and lighter. They will be able to be a better partner or mother. They will be able to go about their day with a newfound sense of energy. None of this is a guarantee. Your body or external circumstances could change, but if your internal environment stays the same, you are still you, with the same emotional frequency and ways of thinking, believing, and perceiving.

This rang true for me when I was going through a tough time in my life. I believed that if I could just move to a new city, that it would solve all my problems. I would stop binge eating, the anxiety would magically disappear, and I would be able to be the person I wanted to be; the person I knew I could be. In telling this to my therapist one day, she looks me straight in the eye and says, "Wherever you go, you take you with you."

Even amidst the "aha moment" that took place in her office that day, it still took me years to disentangle external circumstances from inner happiness. In hindsight, I know I was victimizing myself. I was placing blame on my city for my behavior and habits around my body and food; it sounds insane to even admit that. Although my therapist brought a new way of thinking to the surface, I failed to fully gain consciousness for my internal environment that was creating my reality. According to Jon Kabat-Zinn, "lapses in awareness are frequently caused by an eddy of dissatisfaction with what we are seeing or feeling that moment, out of which springs a desire for something to be different, for things to change."[46] In other words, I was keeping myself unconscious because acceptance meant I had to take full responsibility for myself, and that felt a lot harder and heavier.

Simply changing your external world may not solve anything. To truly experience heightened happiness, doing the inner work is a crucial prerequisite that so many people overlook. In my previous anecdote, I was relying on this new magic city to finally give me permission to evolve into my true self. I believed being transplanted in a new place where I knew no one would provide me the opportunity to be who I intuitively knew I could be. Upon further reflection, I realized the underlying fear was that I still cared what people thought. Given I was still living among a group of people who had known me my entire life, I was scared to change because of what they would think. The new location wasn't the answer—my own permission was. I had to give myself permission to step into a better version of myself. True health and happiness came after I allowed myself to step into my authenticity. First, I had to change the way I was thinking, and this took increasing consciousness— taking a hard, honest look at myself and my thoughts.

If you currently feel stuck in the way things have always been, this could have to do with the way you are fundamentally thinking, which as I have discussed, not only influences your emotions but your state of being too. The first step would be to analyze your lens. Your lens, or the filter through which you perceive everything, dictates your thoughts, which lead to your emotions, which all ties back into your beliefs.

journal:

What do you believe? Put pen to paper and write down your beliefs about your health and yourself. What are those self-limiting beliefs that are keeping you rooted in old patterns that no longer serve you? Examples include, "I will always be unhappy with my body," or something more deep-seated like, "I am not good enough." After acknowledging these beliefs, consider how they have worked to shape your past behaviors and mindset. Can you determine where they came from? Are there experiences or people from your past that have influenced any limiting beliefs? What do you need to do or, more importantly, what do you need to say to yourself in order to let them go?

To put it in context, while working with my life coach and mentor Ellie Burke, the belief of "I am not good enough" surfaced for me. Initially, I was not able to pinpoint where it came from. We tend to repress emotions that are hard and heavy. Due to a bit more digging, I was able to trace it back to the relationship I had with my father, and the fact that as a child, I never felt as if I could live up to his expectations. Given that he was so emotionally distant, it seemed difficult to receive his love unless I achieved to earn his praise.

That's the thing about childhood—beliefs are easily shaped. It could be some seemingly insignificant situation that gets lodged into your subconscious and creates programming. For example, you are coloring in your coloring book and your mom or dad leans over and corrects you, encouraging you to color inside the lines. You interpret that as, "What I am doing isn't good enough," and it snowballs from there. The programming of "must color inside the lines" takes root to eventually influence future behavior, habits, mental tendencies, and choices. The experience could be something more memorable in which you are publicly embarrassed or someone puts you down for the way you look, but the resulting belief is the same: "I am not good enough." You take this thought and you internalize it, and it basically influences the way you view yourself and the world.

This could manifest in multiple ways for different people, but for the sake of this book, let's stick with the realm of physical health and body. How do you think this lens of "I am not good enough" is going to affect your self-esteem and body image, or the way you eat, exercise, and live your life? Because the thought is uncomfortable (whether you realize it or not), your subconscious will attempt to get rid of it. You will act in ways that result in the feelings of "enoughness," or worthiness, or provide you with a sense of achievement.

During my freshmen year in college, this belief played out in a big way. There was a situation in which I felt very left out. I was trying to make new friends, and the transition to college is hard enough as it is. Because I filtered the event through my lens of "not being good enough," I perceived it more negatively than someone who didn't have this belief, and would have allowed it to roll off her back. Spoiler alert: I ruminated over the situation a lot longer than I should have.

It was during this same year when my disordered eating started. In hindsight, I am able to connect the dots. Imbalances in my social life and relationships left me feeling inadequate. Throw in the fact that academically, I now felt like a small fish in a big pond, and my confidence quickly deteriorated. Therefore, I needed to gain a sense of control and achievement in another area of my life, and like most women, this translated into control over food and fitness. When I would have a day of "perfect" eating, or exercise for hours, or reach the number on the scale, then I could feel good about myself. I could feel proud. I could feel *enough*. As I have already mentioned, however, this feeling never lasted very long because the belief was still there, lodged very deeply.

These beliefs affect our daily lives, not just our overall self-image and relationship with food. My self-limiting beliefs still shine through for me, but the beautiful thing about awareness is that when it presents itself, I now know I have a choice to detach from it. It no longer dictates my emotions or actions because I no longer believe it to be true. There is a difference between having a thought and having a belief; a thought turns into a belief when we accept it to be true. Additionally, when some old programing shows up, I can meet it with curiosity rather than attaching to it and allowing it to influence my emotions and behaviors. All I need to do is ask myself a simple question or inquiry such as, "What is that about?" Then I simply quiet my mind and see what answer comes up. Your intuition is amazing at answering these types of questions.

If you would like a more formal training on how to tap into your intuition and develop this ability, Byron Katie offers a powerful practice; it's where I started. Spiritual teacher and author of *Loving What Is*, she created an exercise (appropriately called "The Work") in which you pull apart certain thoughts through simple questioning. By doing so, you debunk "stories" that may be causing you stress (whether about yourself or others). When you are able to notice the noise that pops into your head, you can engage in a self-guided inquiry process to discern thoughts from beliefs.[47]

I frequently guide my health coaching clients to The Work. For example, something I hear often from my clients is, "If I lose weight, I will be happy." As a result, my clients' emotional well-being is attached to a physical outcome. Even if the belief is subconscious, this implies that feeling a sustained sense of happiness will only come after the lower number on the scale and smaller dress size. If you are repeatedly playing this thought in your mind, and you accept it with certainty, it then becomes a belief.

The Work allows you to dig deeper to figure out if it is true, essentially releasing its power over you. Taking this thought of "If I lose weight, I will be happy," can you know that to be 100 percent true? Because so many of our thoughts are dependent on the future or on circumstances that either didn't happen or haven't happened yet, the majority of them can't be said with complete conviction. To learn more about Byron Katie and her teachings, visit **www.thework.com**.

Since our stories tend to be tied to our identities, this work can bring up some stuff. It is uncomfortable to challenge who we always believed ourselves to be; it's why it's called "work."

Ironically, many humans are comfortable with stress and suffering if that state of mind is perceived to be more "normal" than feelings of happiness and joy. If it is what you know, it might be where your mind subconsciously wants to stay. Yet it doesn't have to be this way—you have the ability to choose.

Ask yourself, what are some of the things you are telling yourself on a daily basis, or in the face of certain circumstances, that are causing unnecessary suffering? These thoughts could be about food, your body, your health, or more in the realm of the abstract with relationships or career. This inquiry process can be applied to pretty much any anxiety-inducing thought. Again, it requires both awareness for when these thoughts come up and the ability to unpack them. Until this inquiry process becomes second nature, putting pen to paper and journaling through the inquiry questions can help.

Going through these steps with your thoughts helps get you in the habit of being a more active, objective participant in your life, avoiding those automatic tendencies of your mind. It has you asking the right questions, getting to know yourself, and how you may be standing in your own way. It allows you to face the obstacles (or what you believed to be obstacles) to your happiness. When you no longer place the blame on external situations, you start to feel more empowered; as a result, you will eventually align with a more peaceful, positive self, also known as your intuition, while releasing the fearful ways of the ego.

I have applied this process to many aspects of my life, but I have never witnessed its power so much as I did the morning after my father passed away. Using what I had learned through Byron Katie's The Work, and the inner work on compassion and self-love I had relatively recently developed, I was able to guide myself from a moment of utter grief to a more peaceful place. I even shared this experience in the eulogy I gave at his funeral:

> One morning soon after his death, in a particular wave of grief, the thought of never seeing him again kept surfacing, and I found myself in tears. And it was this thought of never going to see him again that was amplifying that feeling of void, making it a little bit bigger than it already was. And then all of a sudden I found myself questioning that thought. That is something I have gotten in the habit of doing in the past year or so with any negative or anxious thought that arises. I question its truth. And I found myself asking: Do you know that to be true...this thought of never seeing him again? Do you believe that to be 100 percent true? And my mind got very quiet, I stopped crying, and I felt this peace wash over me. And I knew that the answer was no. I believe I will see him again. I have faith in that much.

To be clear, I am not minimizing grief, especially over the loss of a parent. It is a natural emotion, and everyone should have the freedom and the space to grieve. But in that moment of awareness, I realized I had a choice in what I believed. I had a choice to either keep thinking the thought that was causing me pain, or realize that what I was telling myself wasn't even true at all. It wasn't what I believed. It didn't align with that peaceful inner voice. Because I tapped into what I truly believed and found alignment with that inner being, the pain went away.

I hope this helps you understand that these mindset shifts in the general sense can be applied to so much more than the physical body. And if you are someone who struggles with anxiety in general, or it's just day-to-day stress that has you frazzled or caught up in negativity, know that a different way of thinking is possible.

It is important to know that these changes and shifts will not happen overnight. You have experienced however many years (or decades) of a certain way of thinking, believing, and perceiving, so it is going to take some practice. The most effective thing you can do is really get to know yourself and who you are *now*, not letting any preconceived notion of who you were—the main character in your story up until this point—dictate your future behavior and efforts at change. When it comes to change, we humans create obstacles in a couple of different ways.

There is a reason why change can be challenging: Familiarity is much more comfortable. As soon as you try to make a change, your ego senses the new, unchartered territory and will try and tempt you back to what you know—enter old habits and behaviors. The same thing can be said for when you try to shift to more peaceful, loving mindsets. Your ego doesn't like peace and love, as this state of being means acceptance and calm. When you are calm and at peace and not on alert, that is when you let your guard down. When your guard is down, the predator can catch you when you least expect it; therefore, your ego wants to keep you anxious. But know that we no longer live in a world where you can be attacked from behind by a saber-toothed tiger. We no longer live in a world where you need to be watching your back.

Furthermore, from an efficiency standpoint, change requires energy. To stay in a familiar state of being means you are conserving energy. Your human brain is always going to try and conserve energy (another one of those survival tactics). The image we have of ourselves—the identity of "self"—coupled with our beliefs, are not only deeply rooted in the past but are also stable, because to change an *identity*, well, that would just take too much effort. And this is all *subconscious* unless you do the work to become more self-aware. When our subconscious is in charge, we engage in habits and behaviors that support this deeply rooted way of being, even if we *know* on a logical level these behaviors don't serve us.

In almost every initial health consultation I have with my clients, I hear the same frustration: "I know what to do, but I can't seem to follow through with, or sustain, change." Change often comes with resistance, which can arise for many reasons. Perhaps there is a lack of a deep motivating factor (the reason *why* you want to change); maybe there are lifestyle or circumstantial barriers; there could also be a degree of self-sabotage. The latter can show up in various aspects of life, from your physical habits, to your love life, to your career. Again, this is your brain trying to keep you in a "safe" and familiar space. In his book *The Big Leap*, Gay Hendricks defines this clearly through his "Upper Limit Problem" theory. He argues that in consideration of our goals, we all have a ceiling for feeling good and reaching a certain level of success. When we reach it, we think thoughts, engage in behaviors, return to old habits to stay small, or bring ourselves back down to where we were. Not only are we accustomed to feeling fear, pain, and insecurity, but if those are the emotions we are used to, we will prefer them to the positive ones.[48] It sounds backward, but I bet if you think about it, you could find evidence of it happening in your own life. Without awareness and consciousness for what is occurring, self-sabotage and all of the forces I have talked about up until this point, will continue to work against you *just because you are human*.

How to Habit Hack

A tip I often tell my clients is that of "habit hacking." It involves another chance to put pen to paper and bring attention to those habits or old ways of doing and thinking that might be standing in the way of your goals, and your vision of a higher, healthier, happier self. This exercise helps to shed some light, so to speak. Once you can take a step back, observe, and look at the behavior objectively, you will be able to gather information from the behavior and determine which ones are not serving you or your vision. You will be able to ask questions. You can make the mind-body connection, strengthen the relationship you have with yourself, and make the best choice for *you* from there. Remember, I would argue that everything we do, we basically do it to achieve an emotion; therefore, there is always more than one choice you can make to achieve the same emotion, and there is always going to be one that is a more beneficial behavior than the other. On the flipside of those human forces that may be working against you, there is our amazing ability to choose. Every choice is a chance. For the sake of sounding overly dichotomous, a choice either takes you in the direction of your vision of self or away from it.

I love the quote that is often attributed to Austrian neurologist and psychiatrist Viktor Frankl, and believe it to be very applicable. He said, "Between stimulus and response, there is a space. In that space is our power to choose our response. In our response lies our growth and our freedom." Every time you make a choice, there is a thought and then an action taken, but in between the thought and action, there is a pause, and *that* is where you need to place your attention, because that pause is where you will find empowerment. When we are on autopilot, going through the motions, it's easy to just float right through it. But if you stop and sit there for a bit, you will be able to make a more conscious choice. The pause is also the perfect place to ask questions.

Asking questions can be crucial in the process of self-discovery; they allow you to really tune in and build trust for yourself while figuring out what it is you need and want *in that moment.* They also bring you more into the present, knowing that each day is different than the one preceding and the one that will follow. It is not just making the same decisions and doing the same things on repeat because that is what you did the day before. Questions help you get off the hamster wheel and break patterns of thought and behavior that might be holding you back.

Lastly, questions help us to become better analytical thinkers. Ask the questions that will inspire and motivate you to be your best self. Every morning, ask yourself: What do I need to do to take care of myself today? How do I want to feel today? What is going to make me feel good physically? What is going to make me feel good mentally? Why am I feeling off? What is my body trying to tell me? What could I have done instead to have reached a more positive result? See how this works?

Again, this is not about perfection. There will still be times in your life when you make a choice and engage in a behavior that doesn't serve your best interest; that is OK, and I encourage you to meet *those* moments with compassion. Most of the time, however, as you really get to know yourself, you will learn to use your instincts and innate drives for survival to your advantage. Realization and awareness for these mechanisms must come first; to fully understand what is happening both biochemically and energetically will empower you to become more present. From that space is where you are offered the choice between love and fear. Your power to choose pertains to your thoughts, attitudes, energy, perceptions, and actions. Which ones are in alignment with the person you want to be *in that moment?*

When Laura* first walked into my office, I could sense a certain sadness about her. As a single mom of two young girls, self-care had been something elusive, practically described as "impossible" since becoming a mother. In taking care of her children, she rarely took care of herself (both physically and emotionally), and had many stories around the latter, leading to feelings of guilt, shame, and a fear of failure. I was glad when she decided to sign up for my most extensive program, because I wanted our work together to be slow and sustainable. I wanted to take time to get to know the complexity of her path to this point, helping her to unpack what she needed to shed to get down to the core of what she wanted to achieve.

Given that weight loss was one of her goals, we discussed nutrition right off the bat. When I asked her to walk me through a typical day of eating, she didn't even know where to start. There was no typical day; no rhyme or rhythm to what or when she would eat. A self-described "grazer," her meals not only lacked structure but also nutrients. More often than not, she would grab whatever was easiest, which mostly came in the form of packaged, processed food. At night, after putting her daughters to bed, when the isolation of the evening set in, she would binge eat, turning to sugary sweets to numb the negative emotions and mollify the mental chatter. When she reached out to me, she admitted she had reached a breaking point. She felt out of control in most aspects of her life, and it was time to rein it in.

At each initial consultation, I always have my clients engage in a future self-visualization; in other words, I have them envision that they have participated in my health coaching program, and have successfully achieved their goals. When I prompted Laura to describe what this felt like, she responded, *I have more energy, self-compassion, and self-control. I am much more content and motivated in my day-to-day life, and passing along good nutritional information to my children, modeling how to be a healthy person.*

The goal of this exercise was to shift Laura from focusing on what was wrong to what could be possible. The power of belief is important in attaining any goal. In the initial consultation, I also ask my clients to rate on a scale of one to ten their level of belief for achieving their goals. Laura's was a three to four on a scale of ten. If I could get her to really envision it—take a taste of what "success" felt like for her in mind and body—it would plant a seed. I knew getting there would take baby steps and mindset shifts, but I believed she could get there—she needed to believe in herself.

Given that I am a holistic health coach, I typically guide my clients to set goals from a few different angles. With my weight-loss clients, there is always the physical facet: nutrition and exercise. With emotional eating, I try to teach my clients to be more objective with food through the nutritional science behind blood sugar balance and metabolism. Laura's eating lacked structure, and she was showing clear signs of blood sugar mismanagement. Rather than focus on what she needed to take out of her diet, an initial small habit was what she could add in to set up her day for success. She was a big coffee drinker, so I advised her to add MCT oil and ghee (healthy fats) into her morning cup instead of drinking it black. Almost immediately she felt the effects on her hunger and cravings throughout the day, which gave her a feeling of more control. When it came to what to eat for lunch and dinner, Laura knew planning and preparation would be key, so she carved time out of her day to write down recipes, make a list, and go grocery shopping. Over the next several weeks, she slowly "crowded out" the processed foods with whole, *real* foods, and noted that the food that filled her cart completely changed by our final session.

Her deeper work, however, pertained to the mental and emotional side of things: her relationship to food, the binge eating, and ultimately the relationship she had with herself. A past romantic relationship had instilled some limiting beliefs of unworthiness, and she would need to unpack (and eventually drop) those beliefs to align with her vision of better health. In one breakthrough session, she admitted that she felt she didn't *deserve* to feel as good as she had described in her visualization. Not only that, she believed self-care was selfish, especially as the mother of a child with special needs. To lose weight would mean people would take notice and judge her for focusing on her physical body; this belief was creating a powerful block. She was subconsciously holding herself back, even though on the surface, she communicated she was ready to change. I tried to get her to understand that people couldn't possibly hold that judgment yet (since the weight loss had yet to occur), and the only person who was judging her was herself.

When we don't hold a certain judgment about ourselves, any opinion of others loses its power. To drop the judgment she placed on herself would set her free; it would deconstruct the block she carried, which was standing in the way of her vision. Additionally, when she cut the tie that was tethering her to old beliefs from her past relationship, she could take back her power. To be more present would mean she could root down in reality. What was true for her years ago was no longer true, yet she held onto those beliefs as if they were. She had to let go of what was no longer serving her in order to move forward.

What was important for Laura to understand was that these shifts in beliefs needed to take place before addressing her binge eating at night; failure to do so would mean taking a surface-level approach to the habit. That is primarily what binge eating is: a hard-wired, conditioned response in the face of negative emotions, normally toward oneself or a difficult situation at hand. Laura was harboring some tough feelings toward herself and her life in general, from feeling isolated to overwhelmed. Her brain was conditioned to turn to food instead of allowing her to feel. Around and around the cycle continued. The only way to break it? Consciousness—consciousness not only for the habit itself but also for what was driving the behavior.

There were a few different thoughts she needed to prove untrue as well. Through a self-guided inquiry, she brought awareness to those thoughts that were standing in her way. In recounting a night in which she would binge, she got clear on the triggers. It wasn't the content of the thoughts but rather the *chaos*, which she described as a "swirling hamster wheel of emotions, and feeling out of control in all aspects of my life." I asked her, "Is it true you feel out of control in all aspects of your life? Every single one?" After taking a pause to reflect, her answer was no.

This "aha moment" marked the beginning of a shift. Through the powerful process of asking herself the right questions, she could start realizing what was actually true for her *in that moment* rather than holding onto what she thought was true for her in the past. This became a tool she could always use to feel more empowered. This pause is important, and reminds me of Viktor Frankl's quote: "Between stimulus and response, there is a space. In that space is our power to choose our response. In our response lies our growth and our freedom."

If the "feeling out of control" was at the foundation of the conditioned response of overeating (an experience that matched exactly how she was feeling), then she had to get to the root of the issue— the feeling itself—to change the response. When she started to feel more empowered, the behavior began to change. Toward the end of our work together, Laura updated me on the behavior:

> The nighttime eating has been going much better. There was such an emotional component where I felt overwhelmed and isolated. Now I am in a place where I realize that food can't help me achieve what I was looking to achieve (to have those negative emotions go away). I am finding other non-food-related activities instead (reading, journaling, meditating, knitting). I am also in the midst of developing a relationship with my mind; understanding how it operates and using it to my advantage instead. It's scary work, but it was scarier to engage in behavior that was harmful to my health.

Additionally, she disclosed that when she would overeat sugary sweets, she was essentially looking to feel "rewarded" for everything she did in her day. But when she got clear on that thought, she realized that in the end, she didn't feel rewarded at all. To feel rewarded *for her* meant to feel acknowledged and cared for; the food could not provide that for her. Again, digging a little deeper into the behavior she was wanting to change, asking the right questions, and getting clear on the emotions she was wanting to feel gave her the opportunity to take back control of her behavior.

During our final session, while she said no day was "perfect," she did feel more in control. When making choices, she did so from a place of honoring her body; she would think about what was going on inside (both mentally and physically), which she had never done before. She started to prioritize her health and self-care because it became something she valued. She knew that to be the best mom she could be, she couldn't pour from an empty cup, so to take care of herself became tied to taking care of others as well. After six months together, she had lost 20 pounds and gained a new perspective. Most importantly, she felt proud of herself, and although she would no longer have the accountability of working with a coach, she believed in her ability to hold herself accountable.

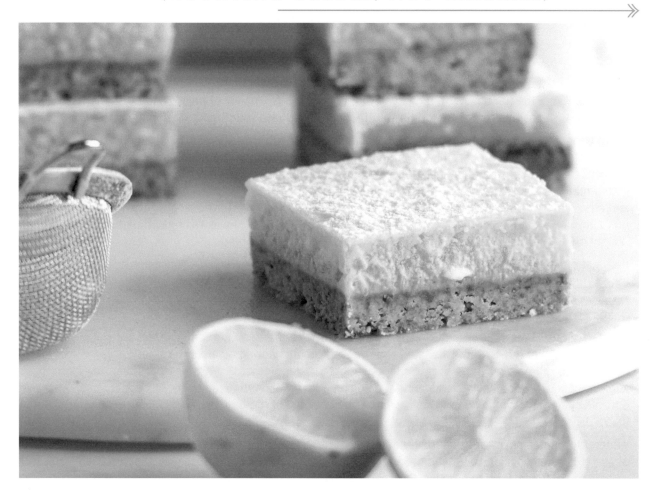

chapter eight:

THE LAW OF ATTRACTION AND MANIFESTATION

*T*his is where the fun begins. You can use your mindset shifts, power of belief, and emotional alignment with positive energy to work in your favor to unfold into your higher version of self.

There was a time in my past when I was going through a difficult time emotionally. In hindsight, I can see clearly that this phase had more to do with my attitude than it did with the external circumstances. In fact, on the outside, everything seemed like it was going swimmingly: I had just gotten married, started a new business with one of my best friends, had good health, lots of friends, and a loving family, but something felt off. Although I didn't know the terminology at the time, I now know I was not in alignment with what I truly wanted for myself. I was letting certain "shoulds" dictate my decisions based on what I was raised to believe that I wanted.

I am not exactly sure where this thought came from at the time (now I know it was an "intuitive ping"), but I felt compelled one day to do a Google search on "uplifting podcasts." To be honest, I had never really listened to podcasts. I don't even think I knew exactly what they were, but this search changed the trajectory of my life.

The Lively Show hosted by Jess Lively was one of the first results. As I started to listen to various episodes, much of the content resonated with me, as she interviewed creatives, entrepreneurs, authors, and self-help gurus. I learned a lot about health, happiness, and business from her subjects, and was soon hooked enough that going on a long walk and listening to *The Lively Show* became one of my favorite ways to start my day (the activity got me into alignment!).

Something I share with Jess Lively is that when we learn something about life that benefits us, we tend to want to share it. I noticed that as she started to embrace the principles of awareness, alignment, flow, consciousness, and the Law of Attraction, her episodes and conversations started to reflect these topics. I had heard of the Law of Attraction, especially in association with the documentary *The Secret*, which I remember watching in college, but the content she was sharing was different. It had less to do with manifesting material objects and more to do with becoming a more present, intuitive, and happy person. Rather than trying to manipulate your external reality, it pertained more to cultivating a peaceful internal experience. The more I applied these principles to my own state of being, the more I witnessed personal shifts in my daily life.

It's important to note here that as far as my external reality is concerned, nothing drastically changed. My mindset, ways of thinking, and beliefs about myself changed, and that was all I needed to take me down a road of inner work. That was when positive shifts started to happen, both internally and externally. As I mentioned, true manifesting isn't necessarily about material things (although it can be); it's about embracing a more positive experience by starting from a good feeling place. It's about changing your lens, unblocking limiting subconscious beliefs, while also aligning with your intuition so you always trust you have the answers you need. It is about understanding that what you want is always connected to an emotion you want to feel, so start feeling that way now to become more magnetic.

In its most simplistic understanding, the Law of Attraction states that "like attracts like." To elaborate, according to Jack Canfield, bestselling author of the *Chicken Soup for the Soul* series and *The Success Principles*, it says, "What you think about, talk about, believe strongly about, and feel intensely about, you will bring about."[49] Based on what we are focusing on, we bring into our lives certain experiences of similar frequency. Your emotions, beliefs, and expectations all work to create your external reality.

Remember when I introduced the concept of your emotional frequency? I want you to think of your frequency like your inner vibration. Whatever emotion you are feeling, your vibration will fall on a scale ranging from low vibration, to a neutral vibration, to a high vibration. Here is where you could really get into the science of frequency and attraction. Our emotions match up with certain brain waves: high beta brain waves being those of stress and anxiety; alpha brain waves being those of presence, mindfulness, and flow.[50] These brain waves then interact with your emotional vibration to create an energy field, which is your point of attraction. I strongly believe that the Law of Attraction plays a role in our individual journeys with physical health and achieving what we are looking to achieve.

In my health coaching practice, I often meet with women who want to lose weight, and early in our conversation, it appears that their inability to sustain their weight loss goals and desired physique has less to do with nutrition and exercise, and more to do with their mindset and belief (or lack thereof) in themselves to achieve their goals. A common thread is their frustration with the weight-loss process in general. They might lose a little weight here and there, but nothing seems to stick. They often feel defeated, discouraged, stressed, and anxious.

As I have explained, these negative emotions—stress and anxiety in particular—alone could be what is standing in the way of feeling your best self. And that theory can be applied to not just weight loss but also low energy and digestive problems. Remember, your physiological inner environment is highly tied to your mental and emotional state. I also want to make it clear that it is not only about the physiological effects of that mind-body connection but also the energetic effects.

This is why I encouraged you to observe your emotional frequency. How would you characterize much of your waking state? Are you present, peaceful, and calm? Or does your vibration fall on the end of the spectrum with more negative emotions, stress, and high beta brain waves? To pinpoint it a bit further, how is your emotional frequency around your health goals? Remember that when we are on a diet, restricting, or counting calories, and worried about what we are eating, that isn't doing us any favors. It keeps our bodies in a sympathetic nervous state with high beta brain waves and lower frequency vibrations. The Law of Attraction then states that you literally can't attract those positive circumstances or emotions you are wanting to feel through goal achievement; it defies law.

You are doing yourself a disservice to struggle your way to what you want. There is a common belief that anything worth achieving takes hard work. We even might have been raised to think "things aren't just handed to you," and the glory comes in the struggle and "efforting" your way to a goal. It doesn't have to be this way, because eventually, your thoughts, fears, beliefs, and lower vibrational tendencies will all come through and keep attracting experiences of similar frequency. If you want a stronger, healthier body because you think you will be happier as a result, but the journey there is one laced with stress and anxiety, you are likely to be very disappointed; in other words, you can't get happy ending from a path that isn't also happy. If you are attaching feeling a positive emotion to an outcome (i.e. feeling happy and more confident to a certain number on the scale), but have yet to get to the root of your dissatisfaction with yourself, the feeling is less likely to last.

I once heard someone say the Law of Attraction is as real as the Law of Gravity; it isn't some new-age phenomenon. It has always existed and you have been using it all along, whether you have realized it or not. Now with a new sense of awareness, you can learn to use it to your advantage.

YOU CAN APPLY THESE PRINCIPLES TO ANYTHING IN YOUR LIFE. LIFE IS ONE BIG JOURNEY.

Try this visualization: Think of life like your floating down a river (on a raft, in a boat—choice of vessel is yours). Are you focusing on your destination or certain conditions that must be met in order to feel a certain way? Or are you enjoying the ride? Whenever I feel out of alignment, this is a mental exercise I play. I picture myself in an inner tube going with the flow of the water, knowing it is natural to come across rocks and rapids, but having the full confidence I will be able to navigate them when the time comes. Life isn't without obstacles, but having belief in yourself to move through them (rather than repress or ignore them) is true empowerment. It is also empowering to know you don't necessarily have to anticipate these obstacles, which can also create anxiety along the way. In this respect, another analogy my life coach Ellie Burke taught me is that of a football player running down the field. He isn't thinking, "Twenty yards away, I will get tackled." No, he is in his body, playing the game, with the confidence that he will pivot when needed as he meets the moment.

If you are riding along the river (or running down the field) of life in fear, anxiety, and negativity about yourself, state of being, and circumstances, the Law of Attraction states you could be attracting lower vibrational situations based on your emotions and beliefs; this can manifest in your physical body. As I have stated, the amazing thing about this is you have the ability to choose your thoughts, create more positive emotions, alter your brain waves, be more "high-vibe," and literally attract what it is you want in life, whether that is better health, a stronger body, or something else entirely.

A major misconception with manifestation and the Law of Attraction is that it mostly pertains to the thoughts you think. Remembering the model that your thoughts lead to your emotions, they do play a role to some extent; however, thoughts alone do not dictate what will show up in your experience. Thoughts will ebb and flow, come and go; it is our attachment to them, coupled with the intensity of our emotions behind them, and lastly the amount of belief for them (which, again, could be lodged deeply in your subconscious) that influence the results in your reality.

Life coach Brooke Castillo says wanting something when you believe you can have it is so much fun, and that [wanting] is only exhausting when we believe we can't have what we want."[51]

This isn't the case when you want something and the way there feels hard, exhausting, painful, and stressful. When you feel positive emotions on the journey of attaining what you want, you will be fueled and motivated by your abundant mindset, and the result will also feel amazing because you will already be feeling good.

Bringing it back to your body and physical health, you can use the Law of Attraction to your advantage. No matter where you are with your current health journey, it is safe to say that we all hold a vision on how we might grow and improve.

Perhaps your goals pertain more to the physical: weight loss, increased energy, improved digestion. Maybe for you it is more mental and emotional: a better relationship with food and less anxiety about whether you are doing "enough" to take care of yourself. Perhaps the way you want to feel has less to do about health and more to do with external circumstances pertaining to your relationships or career. Maybe you are not able to pinpoint the details, but you know that there are better habits you could adopt to feel happier, lighter, and more confident. Either way, you can use your mind, belief, intuition, alignment, and flow to help get you to a better feeling place. Consider everything I have discussed with regard to nutrition, mindful eating, and mindfulness in general; when our bodies are in that sympathetic, lower vibrational state, this has negative physiological, emotional, and spiritual consequences. Practicing presence can provide you with insight into how to achieve your vision.

I want you to start taking the concept of Counting Colors off your plate, and begin to apply this principle to your daily life. Increase your mindfulness not only with your meals but in your daily life as well. Start to witness the beauty around you, knowing that in the moment, everything is as it should be. Noticing the small joys of your day, rather than being attached to the more significant events to drive your happiness, has positive implications for your overall wellness. Looking through the lens of your intuition, tap into the truth of what "is," and allow your observations to be magnified with love and gratitude. You will also be harnessing the emotions of awe and wonder, which studies have shown not only help to foster happiness but also lead to both increased authenticity and prosocial behaviors.[52][53] It can be easier said than done, however; the majority of people have spent most of their time living in their heads, so the mindset shifts and awareness must come first. Then it is a daily practice of noticing and aligning with the present moment. I will be giving you tips on how to more fully embrace the practice.

Using your vision of physical health as a platform to practice, know that when it comes to your "story," and your experiences up to this point that shaped the way you view yourself, your body, your health, and your path, you can let it go—give yourself that permission. You are not your past; release its grip on your present situation, thoughts, and mindset. It will never completely go away because it is a part of you (thank you, memory), so simply use it as information, but detach from it. Learn to process it more objectively. If you are having a difficult time completely letting go of your past, or don't believe you can, simply start with compassion. Have compassion for your past. Both the good and the bad experiences have shaped who you are today. You have developed a certain level of skills and strength along the way; that is something to celebrate.

The concept of letting go can also be a challenging one to wrap your head around. In his book *The Genius Zone*, Gay Hendricks provides an effective visualization exercise for letting go. Imagine holding a ball or other object in the palm of your hand, with your palm facing the floor. Feel the grip of your fingers around the object and the sensations that are required to keep it there; then release it, and let it drop. The tightness you felt in your fingers immediately softens. Then hold the ball or object in the palm of your hand, with your palm facing up. Feel the same sensations, and then release the grip. The object remains in your hand, but instead of holding onto it, you are simply allowing it to be there without attachment. Whether you allow it to drop or allow it to be, the end result is the same: you have let go.[54]

Also learn to discern the difference between your ego fears and intuitive knowing, trust and love. Realize when your ego starts to overshadow your more peaceful intuition—when this is taking place, you can acknowledge it, use it for further understanding of the situation at hand, and tap back into your inner guidance system to take the necessary action steps to get back to a good feeling place. Choose the freedom of not allowing outside circumstances or even your own fearful thoughts to affect your vibration. The practice of mindfulness works to "disrupt the drift"; it slows down the momentum created by your thoughts and emotions, helps you take a step back and become an objective observer, and instills a feeling of empowerment to make another choice or choose a different thought.

I once did a visualization exercise with my life coach. I was going through another one of my "ruts," not able to effectively communicate why I was feeling a low-level, generalized feeling of dread. I closed my eyes, and through her prompts, I suddenly saw myself in my own living room, except I was a miniature version of me trapped inside a small glass box. As I looked around, I saw the routine of the morning unfolding around me: my dog asleep on the couch, my husband in the kitchen making a sandwich. I felt small (literally and energetically) and was unable to use my voice to express my needs. As my life coach continued to walk me through the visualization, I had some major "aha moments." It became apparent that no one was keeping me in this glass box but myself. All I needed to do was break through the walls and stand up. It was a self-created prison constructed by the pressure I put on myself in my work, relationships, and even physical health. The realizations were profound. The pressure still exists, as unlearning this mental tendency is not going to change overnight. I have had over two decades of thinking and perceiving myself in a certain way, but I now know that it is not up to anyone else, or anything else, to liberate me. Freedom comes from the inside. It is an energetic state of being. We simply believe outside circumstances are conditions to make us feel a certain way, and this is the furthest from the truth.

journal:

Give yourself permission to free yourself from the chains of your past. Write down your vision for better health and happiness. In other words, rewrite your story from this day forward because you can. What do you want? How do you want to feel? What do your days, your relationships, your energy look and feel like? Don't hold back—think big. Or better yet, don't think at all. Refrain from using your mind and use your intuition instead. Depending on whether you sense your intuition in your gut or heart (stomach area or chest), put all feeling into that space and write from there.

Remember, you can write the words and even say them out loud, but if you have a goal and you have a vision, if you don't *feel* the emotions first, and you don't *believe* you can get there, there will be resistance. Emotion, or "e-motion," literally means "energy in motion." There is so much energy behind our emotions. They are powerful and deeply wired into who we are, not to mention that our cells can get addicted to certain emotions (more on that in the next chapter); it is why it takes conscious effort to retrain our brains.

All of this sounds good in theory, but how do you do it? Break it down so you can start applying it to your day. An important first step is to bring attention to your thoughts, make the necessary mindset shifts, and tap into more positive vibrations. This is what finding alignment and flow is all about. Alignment is when you are "in line" with more positivity and peace. From that place, you take *inspired action*. Yet give yourself some grace. If you are someone who has been operating at lower vibrational frequencies for a while, you aren't going to jump to elation and joy at the first try. You simply need to shift up on the emotional scale, eventually seated more in a parasympathetic nervous state with slower brain waves. Physiologically, this has such positive implications for your physical body as well, so it all comes full circle.

A good starting point for this work is the beginning of your day: the morning. Your morning sets the tone for the day. Even if you have not realized it, you probably have already experienced the Law of Attraction at work. If you are human, you have had a bad day. Have you ever proclaimed yourself to have "woken up on the wrong side of the bed," and from there it was as if nothing seemed to be going right? You spilled your coffee, you got in a fight with your spouse or partner, you got stuck in traffic on the way to work, and then you opened your email to find your boss berating your latest assignment.

Consider the opposite. You wake up feeling good and the day seems to unfold in your favor: your children are being obedient, you leave the house on time, you arrive at your favorite coffee shop and for some reason your usual latte is on the house, you hit every green light, and get to work and discover you are up for a promotion. These are examples of the Law of Attraction, and your mornings can make or break your day. Bring more awareness into your morning and the momentum you might be creating. What needs to change (if anything)? Can you be better prepared? Can you create more space?

No matter what time I have to be somewhere, I carve out time in my morning for mindfulness. Reading uplifting books, journaling, meditation, and movement are the secret sauce to my self-care and sense of wellness in the early hours. I personally had resistance to meditation for years, but now I crave at least five minutes in the morning; that is all it takes. As I have mentioned, meditation is not about clearing your mind completely, it's about getting to know how your mind operates. It is the practice of gently guiding your attention back to what is real in the moment and with compassion. I will talk more about meditation a little later.

My goal is to help you create more colorful and beautiful days. You do this through mindfulness, awareness, and conscious effort. It does take *consciousness*, but that doesn't mean it is "hard." Our egos and human brains will label something as hard or easy because that is what it is designed to do. As my life coach and mentor often reminds me, the present moment is always a neutral experience. Without the filter of the mind, we are able to peel back the layers to truth—the way we perceive it is up to us.

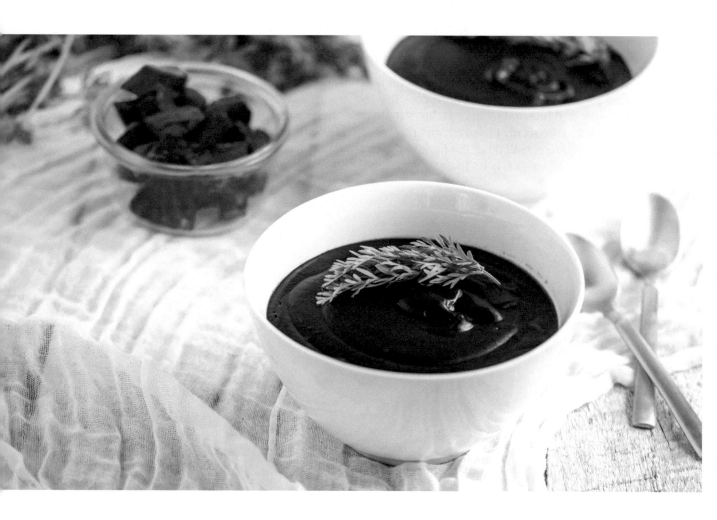

chapter nine:
THE POWER OF BELIEF

*t*he level of belief you have in yourself to achieve your vision (whether for your health, career, love relationships, etc.) can tell you a lot about your subconscious and if there are any blocks still holding you back. In its simplest form, a belief is a thought you keep thinking until you hold it to be true. It can be a conscious belief (you are aware of it) or subconscious belief, meaning it is a thought or axiom instilled in you at a young age by a parent, sibling, teacher, or peer, which became lodged in your mind and influences your choices, habits, and behaviors years into adulthood, even when you are unaware that is what is taking place. I think of this as "programming," a system of beliefs on which you are operating but not necessarily aware of it. Just as a computer is programmed with various software on which it automatically runs, these beliefs work to create your mindset—your "lens"—which has both physiological and energetic effects on your reality.

Consider the power of belief in conjunction with the placebo effect. Numerous studies show that the body's responses to drugs and medications are in part placebo based. Furthermore, it does not just come down to a placebo's deceptive nature or the fact that people think they are taking real medication. Ingesting a sugar pill has been shown to be just as effective as medication when participants are told about a placebo's potential to heal, even though the participants are in fact aware it is a placebo. This is called an open-label placebo trial, and the results are astounding.

Dr. Ted J. Kaptchuk, a professor of medicine at Harvard Medical School and director of the Harvard-wide Program in Placebo Studies, conducted an open-label placebo trial in which he worked with people with irritable bowel syndrome (IBS), which is a pretty common condition that causes a range of digestive symptoms including, but not limited to, abdominal pain, diarrhea, and/or constipation. Half of the study volunteers were told they were getting a placebo and the others got nothing at all. He found that there was a dramatic and significant improvement in the placebo group's IBS symptoms, even though they were explicitly told they were getting a "sugar pill" without any actual medication. The way this works is because not only are they told they are taking a placebo but they are also explained how placebos work and how powerful our minds are. That belief and the power of the mind to "trick" the body into believing it is receiving medication is what leads to results and healing. That pure belief by itself will affect us on a physiological level.[55]

Another fascinating study took the placebo phenomenon a step further. Researchers found that patients with osteoarthritis of the knee that underwent placebo surgery were just as likely to report pain relief as those patients who underwent the actual procedure. The study entailed a total of 180 participants, who were divided into three groups. One group underwent a procedure in which the cartilage was cut away and removed; the second group had bad cartilage flushed out; the third group had the placebo surgery, in which there were incisions of the knee, but no procedure took place to remove the problematic cartilage. Before the study, all participants were made aware that there was a possibility they would be in the group that did not receive the actual surgery, and even wrote in their chart that if they *were* a part of the group that received the placebo surgery, they believed they would not notice any benefits to their knee health afterward; however, the findings proved otherwise. During two years of follow-up, patients in all three groups reported moderate improvements in pain and ability to function. However, neither of the intervention groups reported less pain or better function than the placebo group. Indeed, the placebo patients reported better outcomes than the debridement patients at certain points during follow-up. Throughout the two years, the patients were unaware of whether they had received real or placebo surgery.[56]

The mere possibility that these participants could have received the real surgery was enough to affect them physiologically. Belief combined with expectation is a powerful dictator of results.

When Beliefs and Expectations Combine

Not only do your over-arching beliefs for your body, health, and yourself influence your reality, but the outcomes you expect might just be the results you get.

Mindset researcher Alia Crum reinforces the concept of "what you focus on, you attract," or "the effect you expect is the effect you get."

In his study, Crum recruited housekeepers from seven different hotels across the United States to show how expectations affect health and weight. Why housekeepers? Because housekeeping is physical work, which burns over 300 calories per hour, making it comparable to weight lifting, aerobics, and a fast-paced walk; comparatively, sitting at a desk burns about 100 calories per hour. Of all the housekeepers in the study, two-thirds believed they were not exercising regularly, and one-third stated they did not exercise at all. Not only that, but their physical appearance and test results reflected this belief: they were overweight with high blood pressure.

The housekeepers were split into two groups: one group received a mindset intervention that informed them that their daily work was physically strenuous and should be considered exercise. The second group (which served as the control group) received a lecture about the importance of exercise, but were *not* told their work qualified as such.

Four weeks later, the first group as a whole had lost weight and body fat, had lower blood pressure, and even showed increased job satisfaction with no other changes made to their diet or lifestyle. The housekeepers in the control group showed none of these improvements.[57]

Nothing in their external circumstance changed; it was the mere *perception* of what they were doing and a shift in expectations for an outcome that changed. The lens through which they viewed their job and activity level changed. As a result, they saw changes in their physical bodies.

Rachel* initially reached out to me for help with weight loss, although I realized from just a few sessions with her that there was more complexity to her health journey than simply wanting a lower number on the scale. The scale was the driving force behind her behavior; not only that, but whatever it read dictated her moods. If the number went down, she felt proud and accomplished; if it went up, feelings of shame, disappointment, and failure would follow. But this was not an every-once-in-a-while occurrence—she was weighing herself six times per day.

One of the first things she said was that she "had read every nutrition book out there and tried every diet under the sun" but nothing seemed to stick. I quickly became aware of her incessant negative self-talk. She was "good" if she ate healthy, "bad" if she didn't, and "stupid" if she got off track. Her language was laced with judgment, using words such as "willpower," "guilt," and "cheat" to describe her diet. She was confused nutritionally, frustrated physically, and exhausted emotionally. Rightfully so.

As we went deeper, she uncovered some long-held beliefs she carried about her body, food, her health, and self. One of these core beliefs was that she had always had a hard time losing weight—especially when compared to other people—and that she believed she will always have a hard time. She believed it must be that she lacked willpower (because what's the use?) and how it was "unfair" that others could eat whatever they want, while not gaining a pound, but if she so much as looked at a piece of cake, she would gain five.

We examined her eating through a food journaling exercise. She noted uncontrollable cravings, overeating, food anxiety, and relentless hunger. Her eating rhythms were out of sync, and her cortisol levels were riding high. Knowing that her relationship with food would have to fundamentally shift in order to create sustainable change, I tried to have her look through the lens of neutrality, putting more of a scientific spin on nutrition. To release the language of judgment, and instead put certain foods into categories of either "nutritious" (benefits her physical body) or "not nutritious" (does not serve her physical body). Change in this way was not going to happen overnight—over thirty years of thinking one way takes time to shift—but it was a start. It was important for her to recognize that rewiring new neural pathways takes work to avoid feeling defeated. I explained that the human brain can often be the biggest hurdle, but when she learns to work with her mind, rather than allow it to take over, it can be a powerful thing.

In our time together, Rachel demonstrated some pretty powerful emotions as it pertained to her health and body. Victimization, anger, and shame led to such a sense of separation that learning to work with both her brain and body was going to take some effort. It was also apparent that she engaged in self-sabotage, both consciously and unconsciously, that kept her in the cycle. Ironically, the mindset she had held onto for so long regarding her weight was comfortable; to change how she viewed herself would mean letting go of a part of her "self" (i.e. ego) that influenced how she operated. Even though on the surface she wanted to lose weight, achieve her goals, and embrace a more positive way of thinking, deep down her subconscious was clinging to a way of "being" that was rooted in her identity. Not only that, it was masking some pretty hard emotions associated with difficult life experiences she had gone through in her past.

In one breakthrough session, she admitted to no longer feeling committed. I had her reflect on what commitment felt like. She responded, "empowered, strong, successful." While she said she felt as if she was a strong person, she didn't feel as if she was living in alignment with what she wanted to do with her life: get her business up and going, and be the entrepreneur she knew she could be. She felt angry at herself and her path to this point for not going after her dreams.

She had quite the "aha moment" when I painted her the parallel between the disempowerment she was feeling in the face of her health goals, and that with her life goals. That to feel empowered and confident is a choice—one we can make in the moment—and that there is nothing outside of us (whether it be the scale, a situation, or a person) that can help her feel that way. Victimization can be the easy road to take because taking emotional responsibility for the way we feel is the courageous choice.

From that session on, her health journey became more holistic. While we continued to work on both the mindset side of things as well as tweaking her nutrition to find what realistically worked for her, shining a light on the emotional work Rachel had to do alongside the physical was a game-changer in achieving her goals. After our final session together, she confessed to rarely weighing herself, with her main focus around food being on high-quality meals her body deserves; that her choices were backed by an intention of honoring her body, rather than beating herself up. Even though she lost weight, shifting to a place of self-love was the true transformation that took place. Her beliefs about herself, her body, and what she deserved helped to create that slow, sustainable change she had craved all along. Not only that, she now considers herself the lucky one—that her health goals encourage her to eat colorful food that nourishes her physical body.

Are you starting to realize the role your mind plays in your physical health? To be clear, this is not to say you can forget about nutrition and movement, sit on your couch eating non-nutritious, low vibrational food, and "think" your way to a healthy body. The main takeaway is that if you are someone who wants a certain result (whether that has to do with your health or not), but you don't believe you can achieve it or you are focused so strongly on the "not getting" of the result, then scientific research suggests you might get what you expect.

Remember, you can't suffer or overly stress your way to what you want, whether that has to do with your physical health or something else entirely. You are now aware of how negative emotions may be hindering your health goals from a physiological perspective, but what a lot of people fail to consider is how the negative emotions might be affecting them energetically; in other words, energy flows where your attention goes.

An analogy I often use is that of a couple trying to get pregnant. As a disclaimer, I understand that each couple's path to pregnancy is different, and this will not apply to everyone, but perhaps you have heard a similar story of a couple who has a "miracle baby." After years of trying to get pregnant, they "let go," decide to adopt, or take a break from trying. Soon after, the woman gets pregnant. I know each individual experience is different, but after months of attempting to conceive (without success), emotions can run high (anxiety, stress, frustration, feelings of failure). The focus goes from the joy of having a baby to the *lack* of getting pregnant. Beliefs, expectations, and a woman's inner environment (hormonally and energetically) all shift. I believe this phenomenon played into my attempt to get pregnant with our second child. After six months of trying, I could feel the anxiety build. It was only after I let go, loosened up, and shifted my mindset to more peace and confidence did we conceive. Again, I am not minimizing or discrediting a couple's desire to get pregnant, or the negative feelings associated with the process; it's a complicated topic and, as a human, these feelings are only natural. But these examples perhaps prove that letting go of the pressure has its positive implications.

Why does that happen? The sympathetic nervous state—the one characterized by stress and anxiety—is not the state when your body is in balance. If it is not the state when your organs and biological mechanisms are functioning as they are supposed to, then your body communicates to your brain that it is not the right time to get pregnant. I also believe this example has implications for other issues pertaining to your physical health and to the role that stress, expectations, and perception of "self" play out in your reality.

I encourage you to reconsider your lens. Are you looking through one of lack? Do you feel as if you aren't doing *enough*? Do you believe that achieving better health is hard? Do you believe that your days should be stressful and exhausting? Would you characterize your mindset as negative? If so, that is the type of experience you will have, that is what you will notice, and those are the types of experiences that will be attracted to you.

Karen* came to me for health coaching because she was overweight and looking to lose sixty pounds. As a wife and mother of two young boys, she was also in graduate school part time, earning her business degree.

On our initial consult call, she stated that she had tried many diets with no success, and was craving sustainable change without the stress and anxiety associated with restriction and deprivation that traditional diets entail. Right away I knew we would make a great team in helping her achieve her goals. As the conversation continued, I had the realization that I often do with women who have been on a long journey of dieting. Her lack of success in the past wasn't necessarily about the food she was eating or the way she was exercising (or wasn't exercising); it was more about *how* she was eating and the mindset she had for herself and her health in general.

Karen had a story from very early on in her life that was keeping her trapped in a relentless cycle. After a couple months of working with Karen, she was able to make connections between some of the emotions she was feeling in other areas of her life, and the way this was manifesting in her relationship with food and in her physical body. Deep down, she was feeling lonely, trapped, and disempowered in her life, and that paralleled with how she felt in her body and in the face of food.

On top of that, one of her long-held beliefs was "Life is hard and stressful, and things don't come easily for me," so her journey with food and her weight reflected that as well. During one breakthrough session, she was able to realize that the extra weight she couldn't keep off was a reflection of these feelings, and the belief of "this doesn't come easily for me" just made her feel as if she had to struggle in the process. Because that is what she believed and that was the lens through which she was looking, she was creating that type of experience in her reality.

When I asked about her belief, on a scale of one to ten, in her ability to achieve her goals, the number was quite low; it was uncovered that she really didn't believe things would ever be any different, since this is the way it had always been, and that she would forever find herself in this cycle. And as long as she kept approaching the process from that place, those conditions would keep manifesting in her weight-loss efforts. I asked her *why* she wanted the weight loss and sustainable change; she responded that it was ultimately about feeling free and in control.

As soon as she realized that the feeling was a choice she could make starting in that moment, that she could ultimately free herself and choose to feel in control (because she was), the more she started to feel calmer and more at peace. More importantly, she started to believe in her ability to rewrite her story. The only thing that was keeping her trapped in the cycle was her own mindset around it. She could step out of the role of victim and choose to see things differently. Instead of the weight loss freeing herself from the cycle, she freed herself. Eventually, she saw progress, and she slowly started to see the weight come off.

When you can approach your health, self, and life in general from a perspective of beauty and abundance, this is when you start to see the positive shifts and sustainable change. Although you might not have been raised to think this way, life is supposed to be fun! Not just on the weekends or while on vacation, but when you are truly present, each moment is its own unique experience. I was once having a conversation with my life coach about boredom, and she informed me that when you are truly conscious in the moment, boredom can't exist because every moment is always new; you are always experiencing it for the first time. You simply have to stop and notice the "newness."

Yet we often walk around on autopilot mode, going through the motions; doing things each day tied to a routine because that is the way we did them yesterday. And the day before that. And the day before that. This isn't necessarily living, rather more like operating according to how you were taught to get by: life is hard, life isn't fair, money doesn't grow on trees, you have to work hard to be happy, happiness is fleeting, work is stressful. We have lost sight of what life is about. Really think about "humanness"—why are we here? Is it to constantly worry, struggle, and victimize? Please know that I am not including clinical anxiety or depression in this conversation. If that is something you suffer from, I urge you to talk to a trained professional. I'm talking more about the choice of negativity. Often, this is an unconscious choice, and it can also be habitual.

As I mentioned in the previous chapter, creating more beautiful days can come from your beliefs and expectations as much as from your behavior and choices. When you step out of the paradigm that things happen "to you" in your day, and realize that you can take more of an active part in *creating* your day, your energy and the way your days unfold will shift. So where do you start? I suggest the morning. How you spend your earliest hours, down to the thoughts you think, can set the stage for the type of day you will have.

Positive affirmations in the morning can be a powerful practice. I am going to talk about the benefits of creating more space in the morning in the next chapter, but I want you to think about an affirmation as it applies to you and the way you want to *feel*. Taking your vision for a healthier version of yourself, pinpoint the emotions you want to feel through the achievement of that vision, framing it in a way as if you are already feeling them *now*. From there, come up with a one-sentence statement that basically sums up what you want. For example, "I feel good, confident, and energized in my body," or "I am living in a strong body with a clear mind." Then start to notice the first thoughts that come into your mind the moment you open your eyes. If they are negative, or stuck in a space of dread or victimhood to the external circumstances you have going on that day, say your affirmation, either in your head or out loud. Witness the shifts start to take place!

Keeping your affirmation in mind as your "end goal" (for example, to feel good, confident, and energized), you create your day from there. This affirmation becomes your new lens. Each day you are faced with an accumulation of choices. You have control over a lot more than you think you do, and when you don't have control over something (the weather, what someone says to you, a canceled flight), you can control the way you perceive the situation and the way you respond. Sometimes a situation is not able to be viewed positively, but you can choose neutrality. Accepting the way it is while also acknowledging the elements are beyond your control can be just as empowering and liberating. You will notice a change when you filter your thoughts, perceptions, and choices through this new lens.

Although this is more of a surface-level example, when it comes to food specifically, we humans have control over the food at the end of our fork, and the perception and the thoughts we think while eating. Even if it is not a completely nutritious choice (which is fine), you can choose how you perceive it (remembering how your thoughts and emotions during mealtime affect you physiologically). Essentially, I want you to connect your health habits to something deeper, more meaningful; finding your motivating factor based on the emotions you eventually want to feel. Most of the time, the choices you make with your food will align with good nutrition because these foods nourish your body, but sometimes this is not the case.

Think about when you are out to dinner for a friend's birthday. If you were to go into the dinner under the umbrella of your mantra (to feel good, confident, energized), allowing those emotions to guide your decisions, what would shift? For example, at the end of the dinner, the waitress brings out a candle-topped cake and you all sing happy birthday. Your friend blows out the candles, and the moment is full of joy. The dessert might not be considered nutritious, but if you were to deprive yourself of enjoying the cake, you would not feel good, confident, energized; perhaps you would feel sad and left out, leaving the restaurant with a good case of food FOMO ("fear of missing out"). So you *choose* to partake and enjoy, doing just that—eating "in joy." Knowing that with each isolated instance, you can always bring your mind to the present and to your mantra. That doesn't mean you have dessert every time you go out to eat; maybe next time you are full, and you know that if you were to eat dessert, it would make you feel uncomfortable, hurt your stomach, and ruin your sleep; therefore, *in that moment*, you make a different choice.

To stay aligned with a good feeling place is the name of the game with each choice you make. Your goal isn't to be perfect and it's not to be "right"—it's to feel good, confident, and energized. How does this feeling *feel* in your body? Remember when you wrote down your truths? Your body is a compass. The way you think and perceive something will result in a physiological response. Use the sensations in your body as a tool. According to Eckhart Tolle, "emotion arises at the place where mind and body meet."[58] It's why you have butterflies in your stomach when nervous, your heart rate increases when you are excited, and goosebumps appear on your skin when you feel fear. Your body will tell you when you are out of alignment with your vision and intuition. It feels more like tightness or constriction, rather than open and spacious. Signals of misalignment arise through your physical body and through your emotions. It is one of the reasons why the mind-body connection is so amazing.

Jack Canfield, co-creator of the *Chicken Soup for the Soul* series and author of *The Success Principles*, says that an easy way to get clear on something is to use the "body sway test" as a "powerful tool for accessing your intuition." Similar to how the body compass exercise will provide you with a certain sensation, Canfield informs us that in the field of energy psychology, there is a theory that your body will sway to one side or another based on what is best for you: "When you ask your body questions about what's right for *you*, it will lean backward or forward in response to your queries."[59] We all have this innate knowledge that we can access when making both big and small decisions for ourselves.

Think of tapping into your intuition as the energy of your inner being. Your inner being *always* wants you to feel good, confident, energized. The moment you are out of alignment with this, two things happen: you will experience a negative emotion, and your body with react in some way. Pay attention to that sensation. Determine if you are someone who feels your intuition in your gut (belly) or in your heart (chest). It is not likely that your intuitive knowing will be felt in your mind (head); it is the difference between thinking and knowing. Take a step back and bring consciousness to the moment. Ask the right questions to figure out how you can get back into alignment, *feel* into the answers, and take the action steps from there.

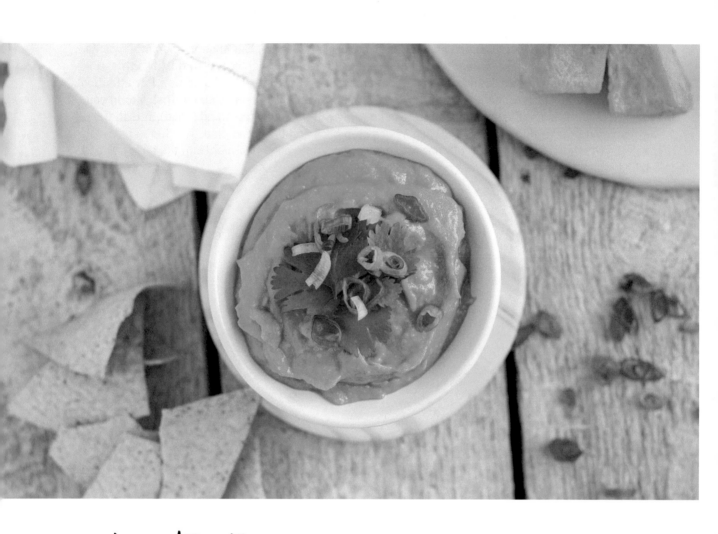

chapter ten:
CREATE YOUR OWN REALITY

Starting Your Day in Spaciousness

The life I've lived thus far feels dichotomous. Thanks to doing this work, I have come to categorize my mindset as "before consciousness" and "after consciousness." The latter can only best be described as feeling more awakened.

Before consciousness (which I also call "before flow"), I would basically wake up anxious, with my thoughts projected onto everything I had to do that day. Immediately, I would be in a lack mentality: feeling as if there was not enough time and then doubting my ability to handle it all. The feeling of dread would rear its ugly head, even before I put my feet on the floor. Given this subconscious belief, it would set me into what my husband called "zoom doom" or "zoom mode." From the minute I opened my eyes, it was "go time." Running on caffeine and adrenaline, I would start checking off the boxes, getting stuff done, just so I could feel good about doing enough. Being enough.

After observing my morning routine, I realized I was creating the momentum of anxiety before even getting out of bed. My mind would race, so to keep up, my actions matched that mentality. I realized I was going through the motions with no awareness, and as soon as I took a step back and began to question, I realized that I was doing this to myself; it was pressure I was putting on myself. To change the momentum, I needed to slow the train enough to hop off and climb aboard another one.

So I slowed down, but it didn't happen overnight. What had to happen first was the awareness for the thoughts that were setting my morning in that hurried motion mentality. As soon as I opened my eyes, my thoughts were: *I have so much to do today. I must do X, Y, Z before breakfast. How am I going to exercise today? What am I going to eat at each meal?* These were the thoughts that contributed to a cloud of pressure, so this mental habit is what I needed to bring my attention to first to start operating in a more positive, loving way. If those self-limiting thoughts occurred first thing, I noticed them, then I would do two things instead, and this is something I still practice: I put one hand on my belly, and one hand on my chest in order to physically feel more grounded, and then I think of three things I am grateful for in that moment.

Next, I reflected on how I would *like* to start my day. In terms of my choices and behaviors, how would I want to fill my time? All I knew was that forcing myself to go to the gym and immediately starting to work afterward was not making me feel aligned; it was only adding fuel to the zoom fire. That was my ego's doing this whole time: making me feel as if I "had to" or that "I should." What my mind and body really wanted to do first thing was feel stillness and peace; that took the shape of journaling, reading, and meditating. I was craving alignment with my intuition. The momentum of feeling good then paves the way for the rest of my day. Most mornings I try to carve out at least an hour for writing, reflecting, and connecting to myself. It doesn't always happen, especially when I am traveling, on vacation, the baby wakes up, or I have an early-morning meeting, but I know it's always there to come back to. If I miss a morning, I don't beat myself up and throw the behavior out with the bath water—I just do it again the next day.

I feel so much better in my body now than I ever did when I was working out intensely, which I believe has to do with starting in more of the parasympathetic nervous state. My inner environment is calmer, my mind is calmer, and my body more balanced. I do still move my body almost every day, but rather than filling my routine with more intense forms of exercise like long stints of cardio, I turn toward hiking in the woods, walking with a friend, and yoga.

Know that it can be easier to stay in alignment and flow on some days more than others, but you will always know when you are out of alignment; your emotions will tell you that much. Your emotions provide you with information. They signal whether you are on or off course. To listen is to take a pause, bring awareness to that pause, ask the right questions, and take inspired action.

If you observe your morning, and find that you are someone who also senses a lot of stress and anxiety, that "zoom doom" I described, it could be time to rethink your morning. Set a new intention. And if setting an intention isn't something you have ever done before, it's time to start! When I talk about segment intending a little later, you will realize that you can break down your day into different sections and set various intentions based on where you are in those moments, for that timeframe, to stay aligned on a more consistent basis.

Maybe you are over there thinking, "OK *Flowy Deschanel*, that's all fine and good, but I have small children and a husband who need to be fed, lunches to pack, a carpool to drive, and then a job to get to or errands to run, and you are asking me to slow down, journal, and meditate in the morning *for an hour*? You have got to be kidding me."

I hear you, so I encourage you to reevaluate your circumstances and ask if there is room to slow down. Are you doing the best you can to create time for yourself? Much of the time it's our stories that create the obstacles to creating space, or making a change, rather than the external circumstances. I often play a game with myself called "Proving Myself Wrong." If there is something I want to do, or a goal I want to accomplish, yet I have this story that creates a reason why it can't be done, I first try to Prove Myself Wrong. The first time I did this was a Sunday afternoon. I knew I wanted to end the weekend eating a nutritious dinner and have healthy food on hand to start the work week, but I *really* didn't want to go to the grocery store. I was tired and making up all of these excuses (It will take too long. The store will be too crowded.). However, I had consciousness for my thoughts, so I played my first round of "Proving Myself Wrong." I timed the trip to the grocery store. Hint: It took one-fourth the amount of time I was telling myself in my mind. Once I was able to fix a healthy dinner and my Monday morning went off without a hitch, I was so glad I went. I have proved myself wrong many times since.

If there is one shift you can do to create more space, honor that. Maybe you can take three minutes to anchor in the moment, check in with your emotions, be in your body, and express gratitude. It really only takes one breath to feel more grounded. If you are someone who loves going to gym in the morning, great! Be sure you feel presence and peace around it. Perhaps you set your alarm ten minutes earlier so you can drink your cup of coffee in peace before anyone else wakes up. My life coach once asked me about something I did every morning that I could use as a trigger to "rest back." Before I drink my coffee, I drink a glass of water first thing. I now associate this habit as a "pause of presence," to rest back in my body and be in the now. What is one thing you always do in your day that can serve the same purpose?

The Power of Gratitude

Having a gratitude practice in the morning is a great way to start shaping a more positive lens. Studies have shown that there is a direct link between thankfulness and overall life satisfaction and happiness.[60] Furthermore, this has implications for your physical health, as people with a daily gratitude practice have reported experiencing more positive emotions, stronger immune systems, and better sleep.[61]

It is nearly impossible to feel a negative emotion and gratitude simultaneously. Try it right now: Think about three things you are grateful for, and then try to feel anxious or sad simultaneously. Furthermore, when you develop the ability to observe and appreciate what you currently have, rather than focus on what's missing in your life, you will feel more expansive and abundant. You also strengthen your "upshifting" skills, teaching yourself to move through neutrality to more positivity. Just as I encourage you to express gratitude before a meal to create more mindfulness, the same can be applied to your morning to create more mindfulness in your day. Consciously feeling gratitude is a practice, and one that creates a foundation for manifesting what you want, whether that pertains to a big dream or the unfolding of a particular day.

The emotions you want to feel are the foundation for manifestation, and then from the place of feeling those emotions—those at more of the positive end of the spectrum—you take action to stay aligned. Ask yourself: What is it you want, and what are the resulting emotions you want to feel? This might change depending on what you have going on that day. For example, on a day when you have to give a big presentation at work, maybe you are looking to feel confident. If you start from a place of gratitude, you can say something like, "I am so grateful for this opportunity to use my voice, creativity, and talents to share my message with my colleagues." If you are vacationing with your family, perhaps you want to feel present and connected to your loved ones. Again, starting from a place of gratitude, count the colors right where you are: "I am so grateful for this time with my family, in this beautiful place, connecting and participating in fun activities." Then think about the action steps and mindset shifts you need to take and make to get there. This allows you to take a step back, *play the whole tape*, shift your focus from the "doing of things" to the "feeling of things," and become more of an active participant in creating your reality.

Default Living Versus Deliberate Living

Many people don't even realize they can be an active participant in their reality. They are accustomed to living their life in "default mode." Default living looks like this:

You have a desire/thought > you take action > you get an outcome > you feel an emotion.

If you are stuck in "default living," you might find yourself on autopilot from the moment you wake up, to the moment your head hits the pillow. You are simply a passive recipient, going through the motions. Things happen to *you*, and you feel the way you feel about them; it's reactionary. Whether consciously or subconsciously, this model puts you more into the role of a victim to your circumstances.

Deliberate living looks a little different:

You have a desired emotion > you get into alignment with that emotion > you take actions > you receive an outcome.

Deliberate living uses the Law of Attraction to your advantage. You are already feeling the positive emotion, and therefore at the vibrational frequency to attract those positive circumstances, and you are in the driver's seat when it comes to creating the experiences you want to have. This is another reason why mornings are so important. You want to create a momentum from a good feeling place to energetically attract situations that are going to reinforce those emotions you want to feel; or additionally, so you start your day looking through the lens of the positive emotion to keep your vibration high.

After expressing gratitude, I encourage you to write an affirmation. Affirmations leverage the power of belief, influencing a more positive mindset. This isn't to say you trick yourself into believing your affirmation, per se—although there might be some of that in the beginning—but remember, the things you tell yourself are so powerful. One thought alone leads to an emotion. Keep thinking the thought and it soon becomes a belief. If you wake up every morning and tell yourself "I am stressed," "I am tired," "I am unhealthy," the resulting emotions and momentum created will be negative, and rightfully so. If you can start to turn it around, using thoughts, beliefs, and the power to choose your emotional state as a springboard for the rest of your day, you will notice positive shifts.

An affirmation is a statement about you and how you want to show up, feel, or be, but in the *present* tense. You prime your brain to start building this belief now, and then that is the lens through which you start to view yourself, your energy, and your state of being. The more consistent you are with reciting your affirmations, the more it becomes ingrained, and it transitions from being a thought to your truth. You start to embody and embrace your new beliefs. Some examples of affirmations are: *I am feeling healthy and strong; I am feeling happy, connected, and in love with life; I am energized and confident in my own skin; I am handling anything that comes my way today.* The affirmations can be different each morning depending on what is going on in your day or life, or they can be the same each time if shifting your fundamental views for yourself is your ultimate goal.

To take this practice a step further, you can turn your affirmation into an intention; this can be very empowering. To put an action step behind your affirmation provides evidence of alignment with your new belief. If your affirmation is along the lines of *I am feeling healthy and strong*, an action that aligns with that belief could be scheduling a thirty-minute strength-training session. Or if you say to yourself, *I am feeling happy, connected, and in love with life*, reaching out to an old friend to go on a walk or grab coffee might reaffirm that belief. Not only does this affirmation exercise put you in the driver's seat of your choices but it also works the other way, helping you to consider whether a choice will align with your desired feeling. Telling yourself that you feel healthy and strong, and then going through the drive-through for a breakfast biscuit doesn't align. The feeling comes first, which then influences your behavior.

Retrain Your Brain Reflection

At the end of the day, you can do something similar, and what I like to call a "retrain your brain reflection." Remember, as humans, we are hardwired to focus and expect the negative. It's a survival defense mechanism, but we no longer live in a world where you have to constantly be watching your back for the big wild boar or saber-toothed tiger, so again, give yourself permission to let the unnecessary anxieties go.

In the evening, or before you go to bed, acknowledge the beautiful, positive, and *colorful* things that occurred, no matter how small or seemingly insignificant. If it made you feel joy, even for an instant, take note; these joyful moments are meaningful and make up the pearl necklace of your life. Maybe you met a cute puppy on your walk or caught up with a friend over coffee. Perhaps it was something larger like landing a promotion. As you start to write down the positive moments, your brain will start picking up on these moments as they are taking place, leading you to feel more present and positive *throughout* your day in the actual experience.

The retrain your brain reflection also helps you take responsibility for your actions, should you react in a way that you wish you hadn't or made a choice that did not serve you. Because you are human, you will likely have days like this; that's OK, we all do. Sweeping change doesn't happen overnight, and your lens may get muddied from time to time. This end-of-the-day exercise is an opportunity to reflect on how you could have done things differently or what you could have perceived more positively. To be clear, this isn't harping on the past; this is coming from a place of empowerment. There is a difference between this reflection and asking yourself, "What more positive thing could have happened to me?" (for example, it could have been sunny rather than rained so my outdoor cocktail party wasn't moved inside). When it comes to this reflection, you want to keep it in the realm of your control, allowing you to take responsibility for your actions, reactions, and emotions.

Taking responsibility for your emotions takes courage. Whether pertaining to a particular circumstance or generally in life, it can feel easier to play the victim. When you aren't responsible for the way you act, think, believe, and feel (meaning you don't have any control over any of it), no other action needs to be taken, and you can coast along doing things the way you have always done them. To your human brain, this is technically easier, because change is more difficult; it takes more energy. Your brain wants to stay on the path it has already paved for itself. To pop out of its current neural pathways and carve new ones would be less efficient. This is why it is encouraged to take baby steps to change, but you first must acknowledge your responsibility and the role you play in creating your reality. You are responsible for your emotions; your emotions, for the most part, revolve around your choices, whether that is in the conditions themselves or in the thoughts you think.

Sometimes you may feel an emotion and not be able to pinpoint why. What consciousness allows you to do is name the emotion, and if it is uncomfortable, and you don't want to stay in a negative space (which, believe it or not, many people do), you do have a choice to get to a better feeling place. You have the power to get back into alignment. When I talk about the emotional scale a little later, you will understand that it doesn't mean you force yourself to feel joy if you are frustrated or angry. It could mean upshifting to more of a neutral emotion, from anger and frustration to contentment. Perhaps petting your dog, going for a walk around the block, drinking tea, and reading a book for ten minutes will get you there. That is all in your capacity of choice.

As you train your brain to catch these instances, the more "in the moment" awareness you will have. Journaling, curiosity, and asking the right questions are all practices of getting to know yourself; getting to know the way your brain operates to determine habitual thought patterns that may not be serving your vision of your healthiest, happiest self.

Meditation or a spacious breathing exercise is another way to get to know yourself and your mind. Many people have resistance to meditation. Whether they use the excuse that they are too busy, don't have enough time, don't have the right space, or are worried they don't know how, I would argue that it's mostly because bringing attention to thoughts and emotions is very uncomfortable. There is a research study that shows 67 percent of male participants and 25 percent of female participants would rather shock themselves than do nothing and be alone with their thoughts.[62] It is why humans often engage in behaviors to numb or ignore the noise in our minds. Why would we meditate to focus on the mind *on purpose*?

I used to feel this way as well. It was exactly why I would wake up and go immediately into "zoom" mode. My morning routine worked to rinse away the negative thinking and self-imposed pressure that became present as soon as I opened my eyes. After I realized I no longer wanted to feel this way (in the morning or otherwise), I took responsibility for my emotions and knew that for something to change, I had to do things differently. My life coach is also a meditation teacher, so with her encouragement, I began incorporating the practice into my day, starting with two minutes, and eventually increasing it to twenty. I now have a meditation space in a bright corner in the back of my house, but it did not start out this way. When I started, I would move a couch cushion to the middle of my living room, sit down, close my eyes, and breathe. Disclaimer: You don't need twenty minutes, and you don't need a pillow, altar, or incense. You simply need a breath (which you have) and the ability to pay attention to it (which you also have). So many people complicate something that is supposed to be spacious, not create more stress.

When I stopped thinking that meditation had to be about clearing my mind completely (because if I couldn't do that perfectly too, why do it?), it took the pressure off of the practice. Your mind will wander, it's what makes you human, and will only stop wandering when you are no longer alive. Meditation is about strengthening the ability to notice when it does, and then gently and compassionately guiding it back to what is real: the present moment, your breath, the sensations in your body.

I have come to crave this moment in my day. I also now know that it is called a practice for a reason. Not only is there no need for perfection, but "practice" also implies something we continuously need to work on. We also don't need to be sitting on a pillow to practice. Meditation can occur when you are driving your car, going for a run, and, of course, fixing your meals or eating your food. It's simply about awareness for the present moment. At a minimum, when you wake up in the morning, put one hand on your heart and the other on your belly. Pay attention to your breath for ten seconds. From a brain chemistry perspective, this is a practice of slowing down your brain waves from beta to alpha, and getting your frequency aligned with the "flow state," making you a recipient (or your point of attraction stronger) for more situations of flow. I will discuss "flow" in more detail a little later.

Increasingly becoming an observer of your mind makes you more compassionate toward yourself. Think of your noisy mental chatter like a toddler throwing a tantrum. At first you want to throw your hands in the air, get frustrated, and urge them to be quiet. The more you keep watching, however, you start to see the humor in the situation; the "humanness," so to speak. The toddler's behavior becomes kind of funny and cute (I know this doesn't happen every time, but bear with me). They don't even remember why they started throwing a fit in the first place, and frustration and irritation get replaced with love, compassion, and empathy. I currently have a toddler, and when I can overcome the initial impatience when he throws himself on the floor and starts crying uncontrollably, I soften and am able to disengage the situation more effectively. Same scenario for the tantrum in your mind: When you notice, catch yourself, and disrupt the drift; this allows you the opportunity to show yourself some compassion, and guide your mind back to the present moment, the only thing that is real.

Using the Law of Attraction to Your Advantage

Developing more self-compassion and self-love has positive implications for using the Law of Attraction to your advantage. The Law of Attraction states that "like attracts like," or in other words, we attract or bring into our experience people and circumstances of similar vibrational frequencies. When you want something but are not an energetic match for it because you are wanting it from a place of lower emotional frequencies, those are the type of conditions you will attract. If you bring your attention to something that you want, does your "wanting" feel like a desperate *need*? Does it feel like an anxious hunger? A holding on too tightly to the idea of it, or an attachment to the outcome without any reverence for the process?

Using the theme of health weaved throughout this book, if you have an idea of your vision for how you want to feel physically, but the journey of trying to achieve it feels desperate and anxious, and you are focusing on the fact that you haven't yet attained what it is you want, you will keep attracting the condition of not having the thing, or the body, or the state of being. The universe always says yes to what you focus on. By focusing on the lack, you will keep attracting the lack.

Ironically, by focusing on the *not* wanting of something, you will still attract it. The quote, "To worry is like praying for something you don't want" sums this up perfectly. However, when you approach your goals and daily life from the positive emotions you are wanting to feel first (by attaining the thing or condition that you want), you will attract the experience or condition because you will be an energetic match for it.

I once had a health coaching client tell me that once she achieved her weight-loss goal, she would feel more "free," "vibrant," and "confident." She said she would be able to go out, enjoy herself, go shopping without shame, attend dinners out with friends without worry, take trips with her husband, and leave the anxiety behind. We talked a lot about the Law of Attraction during that session. I asked her what she was waiting for—feel those feelings *now*. Do those things *now*. Live as if you have already achieved your goals, and the joy and happiness of living the life you want to live can work to attract the vibrancy you want to feel in your physical body.

The reason I believe it is so important to feel the higher vibrational emotions first is because I have experienced the other way around. I, too, once had the belief that if I achieved my goal weight, I would feel similarly. And then I did, and the destination became replaced by a slippery slope. Not only did I continue to feel anxious that the weight would creep back on, but I kept wanting a lower number. I now realize that this was in part due to my inability to get out of the habit of being in a weight-loss state of mind, fighting for the ephemeral "happiness" that comes with seeing a lower number on the scale. I also realized that the story I was telling myself that a lower weight would lead to increased happiness didn't even hold true, so what was I struggling for? True contentment came only after I released both the habit and the old belief (and found my happy weight, which I have maintained for years).

I am not going to sugar coat it—to do this work and rewire a more positive neural net does take effort. It takes *consciousness* and the moment-to-moment awareness I have been encouraging since early on in this book. It is why I introduced it in association with your meals, knowing a meal can be the perfect microcosm of mindfulness, not something to battle with multiple times per day. Meals offer the perfect opportunity to practice *counting colors*, becoming more positive and tapping into a very sensory experience, which is a gateway to the present.

This work takes effort and consciousness because studies have shown that your physical body and mind can literally become addicted to certain emotions as you would a substance or behavior.[63] It is why rewiring new neural pathways in your human brain can be hard. I don't just mean on an energetic level of victimization, staying in a negative space because it feels easier and validating; I also mean on a *cellular* level, with the various neuropeptides that are released in response to the emotions that are felt.[64]

Let's look at what happens on a cellular level when you feel a feeling. When you have a thought that creates a certain emotion, a neuron is fired based on past experiences. For example, say you were bitten by a dog when you were little and developed a fear of dogs. Every time you saw a dog, even years down the road, the feeling of fear would come up for you due to biochemistry and memory.[65] The dog creates an associative trigger and results in a bodily response. These neurons send a signal to your hypothalamus, which is a small cluster of neurons and responsible for many biological functions, especially in connecting your nervous system to your endocrine (hormonal) system. This control center of the mind-body connection explains why you can't separate emotional health from physical health and vice versa. It is a built-in part of our biology. A neuropeptide is then created. This small protein travels throughout the body and locks into your cells, activating a physiological response. Using the example above of feeling fear, you then might experience goosebumps on your skin or an increased heart rate.

Once you are in this state, your brain likes coherence or "sameness," so thoughts immediately arise to reinforce the physiological response. Much of the time these thoughts are automatic and subconscious, but all the same, your mind is receiving the memo that you are feeling fear, your body continues to support the thoughts, and a cycle ensues.

Have you ever had an anxiety or panic attack, or more like a meltdown, and it seems you can't help the negative emotions from snowballing? It is the downward spiral of this cycle that is occurring. Yet what is fascinating and important to understand is that your body and cells could have become addicted to these emotions; or more scientifically speaking, addicted to the protein—the neuropeptide.[66] To clarify, this doesn't mean the way you feel is out of your control, but it is evidence that your old, limiting beliefs and ways of thinking and perceiving are harder to rewire than just changing your mind. It takes conscious effort and awareness. You must bring awareness to the moment in which you find yourself in the beginning of that cycle, and choose a different pattern. The more you practice making a different choice, the more you are rewiring and rooting new patterns.

An example of this happened to me as I was writing the online program version of Counting Colors. I spent an entire Sunday creating the content—six hours straight to be exact. Throughout the writing process, I was backing up my files on a flash drive. When I went to save a full day's work, I replaced the wrong document, selecting the previous day's document instead. Just like that, my whole day's effort was lost. Poof! Gone. To say that I panicked is an understatement. What unfolded in the following five minutes was not pretty. To paint you a picture, I crumbled to the floor crying, holding my head in my hands. My husband came running in as if someone had died. Again, I am not proud of my reaction, but in this experience, thanks to all of the work on consciousness and awareness I had underwent, something happened that had never happened before. After about a minute, I "woke up." I snapped out of it, so to speak, and observed myself from more of an objective perspective. It's almost like I was above my body watching this tantrum take place.

Although I was still amidst a downward spiral of negative emotion, I had awareness for what was happening. The thoughts running through my mind were creating very negative emotions, and as a result, I was experiencing physiological symptoms that then reaffirmed the stories I was telling myself: *all of that hard work for nothing; now I am never going to finish the material in time; I will let everyone down who already signed up for the program; I will likely have to cancel the course altogether.* I think at one point I was literally on the floor pounding my fists. As I watched this taking place, I started to feel something else: curiosity. Being curious for *why* I was acting this way led me to the conclusion that the only reason for my reaction was to feel relief and get what I wanted.

A situation such as this one is an example of how our past programming can manifest. Something subconscious made me believe that if I acted this way—if I cried and yelled and begged hard enough—what I wanted would be on the other side.

I stood up and stopped the spiral. Bringing awareness to the experience helped me realize what was real: My lost file was not on my living room floor. Freaking out was not going to make the file magically reappear. Strong childhood programming probably taught me that a tantrum helped me get what I wanted. Prior to having this level of consciousness, I would have likely kept panicking, allowing my negative emotions to completely paralyze me into inaction, preventing logical thought and reasoning, and allowing this experience to ruin my week. Perhaps I would have even canceled the course, allowing my thoughts and the stories I was telling myself about the situation to manifest a different reality.

In disrupting the drift down to a dark place, I was able to use my pre-frontal cortex to confront reality and empower myself to take the necessary steps to find a solution. What I wanted was the information back, and the only way I was going to achieve that result would be to sit down and produce it. I had to have faith and trust myself that if I could create it before, I could create it again. So that is what I did, and everything turned out fine. I envisioned the result first, the emotions I wanted to feel through achieving it (relief and peace), and I unfolded from there. In these types of experiences, there is always a lesson to be learned. When you find yourself in a spiral, or in a state of being in which you do not want to stay, how can you do things differently that will better serve you?

The ability of your body to get addicted to certain emotions can have a more profound and generalized effect on your life. Growing up, my household was not always happy. I experienced an underlying sense of anxiety throughout my teenage years, although I don't think I could have described it as anxiety at the time. There was often this uncertainty associated with not knowing the mood or energy of the environment I would return to from school. Sometimes there was this sense of walking on eggshells to avoid stirring the pot.

I later made the connection between feeling anxious growing up and the start of my food anxiety and disordered eating freshman year of college (the breakthroughs and "aha moments" never seem to cease when you are doing this work and always learning!). I was out of my parents' home, and I believe my mind needed something else to attach to; something else to be anxious about. I was worried about school work as well, but working hard and getting good grades had always come easily to me. Very subconsciously, I feel as if my brain and body used food and a fear of weight gain not only as the distraction and safety blanket I discussed earlier, but also as a subject to satisfy a craving of these negative emotions I was so accustomed to. Dr. Joe Dispenza calls this "memorized chemical continuity."[67] My body was accustomed to anxiety, and together with my mind, I was creating a reality that "allowed" me to continue to feel it. While I have made great strides to reduce these anxious thoughts, they still show up. Consciousness allows me to know what is taking place and to detach from there and get back into alignment with a more loving energy.

This is true empowerment: knowing you have the ability to use your brain and belief system to create your reality, and to (re)write your story from any point. Mindfulness and presence can help you discover what you need to know or do. Experiences are information to influence your evolution to a more whole, authentic, peaceful person.

Another way to get back into alignment is by creating the positive emotions through aligned action. What makes you feel happy? What makes you feel in the flow? What gets you into alignment so you feel a positive emotion?

Spiritual teacher Gabby Bernstein says, "become a yes for what you want." Make feeling good a priority through inspired and aligned action. When you need to shift toward more positivity, let go of what you think you "should" be doing in that moment, and allow for what feels flowy and unforced.

Ask yourself: When do I feel most in the flow? What makes me feel aligned, happy, and having fun? Write some things down, and see if you are incorporating any of these activities into your day. Maybe it's going on a long walk, or putting on your favorite song and singing, or petting your dog, or doing yoga. A couple of things that make me feel in the flow are when I'm doing food photography, baking, or listening to a podcast while on a walk. Any time I feel like I am out of alignment or in a bad mood (we are human, there will be bad days), I try to stop what I am doing, and do one of these things to get back into alignment. If I am short on time, I know being with my dog for just three minutes is all it takes to increase my vibration, even just slightly. Then from that place of alignment, I will carry on with the rest of my day. Sometimes this is easier said than done, as the mind will come up with excuses for why you don't have time to simply stop what you are doing to do something else for the mere pleasure of it; but trust me, your overall productivity will be better off. The trick is to give yourself permission.

Use curiosity and the power of asking questions to your advantage. Here are some of my favorite questions:

What would make me feel aligned and happy right now?

How can I make this more fun?

What would feel like the least amount of "efforting"?

What do I want to do instead of what do I think I should do? (honesty, authenticity)

Have I been here before [in this emotional state] and did I get through it? (the answer is always yes because here you are, having survived said emotional state).

What can I control in this situation or circumstance?

To clarify, I am not encouraging you to ignore negative emotions or sweep them under the rug. It is about getting out of victim mode, out of being a passive recipient to your emotions, and feeling empowered to choose a different path. We are not the stories of our pasts, nor do we have to stay in them. The beautiful thing is that you can start right now. Every "now moment" is an opportunity to change and shift if needed. We only ever have the present moment, so it's about approaching it with the mindset that it will unfold in your favor. The world and your brain and your body are not out to get you. You and your body are a team with the same goals in mind. Remember, life is supposed to be fun.

Find Your Flow

Food anxiety is a major hindrance to finding flow. In my health coaching practice, I often address the topic of food anxiety with my clients. Food anxiety used to rule my mindset through every meal, so I know firsthand what it feels like. Thankfully, I have come to accept this confusion as part of my past, and it rarely rears its head, yet I also know people (especially women) continue to struggle with it.

Food anxiety is a clear signal that there is a lack of presence in your life. If you are thinking about food during times when it is not on a plate in front of you or when you are planning and preparing your meals, then this is the epitome of not being present. I would even argue that food anxiety plagues one's ability to live fully. Being ruled by ruminating thoughts about food (again, something that you need multiple times each day) prevents you from showing up as your happiest, healthiest self. I will also discern the difference between food anxiety and worrying what to fix your family for dinner. As a busy mom, I know there can be those thoughts of "What are we going to have for dinner tonight?" and that is not what I am referring to. I'm talking about worrying about food from more of a disordered eating standpoint.

Back when my disordered eating was at its height, I thought about food constantly. I had so much fear around food, wondering if I was eating too much, was this food going to make me gain weight, tallying up the calories I had consumed already, and how much I still had left to spend. To make matters worse, because I was always thinking about food, this incessant thinking made me constantly hungry. Remember, digestion starts in the mind, and what you focus on, you draw energy to. I never felt satisfied. I was basically making my worries a reality.

I was always concerned about my next meal or snack: Where would it come from? Would I have something on hand when my blood sugar sunk too low? Hunger and I were not friends, and I was scared of that too—fear being the key emotion. I was definitely not in the flow or happy, for that matter. When I look back on it now, I imagine how much mental energy I could have saved with all of these tools and mindset shifts I have discussed thus far. Unlike other forms of compulsive behavior or addictive thought patterns (substance abuse, shopping, or gambling, for example), a person cannot fully escape food. It is not something someone can abstain from or quit "cold turkey." Quite the opposite. We need it to survive, and are forced to face decisions around it, and the consumption of it, multiple times per day; therefore, it is not something we can run from, so the solution is in establishing inner peace around food.

Additionally, if I had known back then what I know now about the nutritional science behind blood sugar balance, I could have found food freedom a long time ago (to learn more about blood sugar balance, check out my online course: The Beauty of Blood Sugar Balance, **www.balancedbloodsugar.com**). Blood sugar balance coupled with a more positive mindset and relationship with food, *plus* the ability to be more present and mindful, while understanding the way your mind works, is a game-changer.

If you are currently experiencing anxious thoughts around food, apply all that I have been talking about in order to move through them and let them go. Take a step back, bring your mind to the present, and ask questions. Approach your mindset with curiosity rather than with feelings of guilt and shame. What is going on that is causing you to have these thoughts? Ask yourself: Am I physically hungry (stomach is empty and rumbling) or is it hormonal hunger (blood sugar is low, felt more in the head)? Are the worries I have around food and eating real, or am I creating stories in my mind that aren't even true? What am I trying to distract myself from? Are there emotions I am suppressing that I need to give myself permission to feel? Will I eat again (the answer to that question is yes) and will I be OK (the answer to that question is also yes)? What am I doing in this moment that I can bring my attention to? Put pen to paper, tap into your intuition, and see what comes up.

Food anxiety could exist for you for several reasons. It could either be emotional (stems from fear) or more physical (mismanaged blood sugar and hormones). If it is the former, it is then about getting clear on where that fear comes from and what it represents. Using the self-guided inquiry process with those fearful thoughts, start to determine what is real and what is "story." Understand as well that food anxiety and a need to control food comes from some underlying negative emotions and beliefs. As women, it is one of the main things we want to focus on when there is a source of discomfort and imbalance in another area of life. It is something tangible we can control and manipulate. Lastly, when you work on becoming a holistically happier person with a more positive mindset, this shift simultaneously works to reduce your fearful and anxious thoughts around food.

Thinking about food, worrying about your body, and worrying and anxiety in general are clear signals that you are out of flow, out of alignment. Flow and alignment come from connecting to your intuition and being in the present moment. Your intuition knows no fear; it only knows love and peace. In fact, the eternal present, when you fully drop into it, is pure peacefulness.

What exactly is flow? It's that feeling you get when you are entirely immersed in the present moment, a creative project, or a joyful experience. Artists feel it when they are painting; chefs feel it when they are cooking; mothers feel it when they are playing with their children; adrenaline junkies feel it when they are jumping out of airplanes; yogis feel it when they are in warrior two. When you are fully present with one point of focus, the noisy mental chatter fades away.

Studies have shown that people are so much happier when their minds are not wandering. One Harvard study showed that people spend roughly 47 percent of their waking hours thinking about things other than what they are doing in that moment, and that this makes them unhappy. In looking at the data even further, the researchers concluded that the inability to be present was the cause of their unhappiness, not just a consequence of being unhappy.[68]

According to author, yoga teacher, and meditation expert Tiffany Cruikshank, the mental chatter means we lose our sense of flow, which she defines as "the total absorption in our tasks that research has proven is a potent source of happiness."[69] Additionally, unless we are consciously aware of those thoughts that take us out of the present, we may then become bombarded with the many judgements and stories we have around those thoughts. Those stories that are not true, that are rooted in fear, that are centered around the past or future, that create those negative emotions, instigate that downward spiral, and propel us in the momentum to keep attracting lower vibrational thoughts and experiences into our lives.

How much of your day are you currently spending "in the flow," and how much are you on autopilot, just going through the motions and not being fully present in your life? It's like the sensation when you are driving, and suddenly you have arrived at your destination but you can't even remember the journey.

Of course, some things in your daily life must be routine and habitual; it is how your mind conserves energy.[70] If we were to tune in to every single little detail in your day, you would become overwhelmed with information. However, there is a difference between sleepwalking through life and present awareness, which can help you embrace a more positive mindset, seeing and noticing the small things, counting more colors, both sensorily and metaphorically—which can be so beautiful. Because let's face it: Day-to-day life can feel mundane if we allow it to just unfold without paying attention. When you change your lens and increase your awareness for what is, that is when you start to notice more positivity. That is when you have the sensory experiences and see the beauty around you that adds so much to your everyday life. That is what leads to the gratitude and appreciation and positive emotions that solidify the foundation on which you need to proceed with your health goals. As you turn your attention to the positive, what you appreciate *appreciates*. Where your focus goes, energy flows.

On the other side of this coin is the realization that you are still human. You will have negative thoughts and emotions in the future. Your mind will wander, you may react in ways that don't serve you, and you will lose your sense of presence. The important thing is knowing you always have the tools to notice when it is happening, and gently guide your awareness back to the present, doing what you need to do to get into a more positive headspace.

Segment Intending to Create More Flow

To create more flow throughout your day, I encourage setting intentions, not only for your whole day but also for different segments of your day. Daily intentions can be wonderful, but sometimes as we are moving throughout the day, we can lose sight of the bigger picture, especially when we get immersed in our routine settings (work, errands, carpool). Habitual ways of thinking, doing, and reacting click back into place. Setting different intentions for different parts of your day can help with increasing awareness, presence, and flow, from moment-to-moment or segment-to-segment.

For example, a typical day for me can be broken down into my early morning at home, the time spent working on my business, my lunch break, my afternoon (whatever that entails), and my evening, whether that is spent exercising or eating dinner and connecting with my family. Sometimes I even break it down further: my drive to wherever I am going; my daily movement or walk with my dog; the individual meetings, calls, appointments, and desk work; and my individual meals. Whatever it may be, I set an intention for each chunk of time.

These days, it is rarely action-oriented. I used to focus more on my list of to-dos and the boxes that needed to be checked: responding to emails, starting a project, having a call. I shifted my intentions to encompass how I want to *feel* and the necessary steps I need to take to achieve those feelings. During my drive to whatever I have first thing, I want to feel happy, so I turn on my favorite playlist or podcast and try to notice three small things that brighten my day. During my lunch break I want to feel totally present and eat mindfully, so I shut down my computer and put down my phone. During a meeting with an employee or other business professional, I want to feel confident and enthusiastic, so I sit up straight, look her in the eye while I am talking, and make sure she knows I am truly listening. In other words, what is the energy you want to give off. What is the frequency you want to embody? What is it you want to manifest in that span of time?

The segments can be expanded to encompass a weekend, an event, a trip, or a vacation. It helps you tap into the deliberate living I referred to earlier. It's a type of visualization exercise for various blocks of time. You see yourself within these segments, you imagine how you want to feel, and therefore you not only attract circumstances and experiences that align with that feeling, but you also feel empowered to act in a way that aligns with this vision. Do you want to feel happy and healthy during a weekend away with your family? How do you need to be and act to attain that feeling? Better yet, I often have my clients describe and visualize how they want to feel on the other side. Come Sunday, after a weekend away, are you tired and irritable because your trip threw you off track, or are you rested and happy because you enjoyed yourself while maintaining self-care? What are the behaviors and habits you must keep in mind to achieve those feelings? You are basically setting your dial or frequency to this feeling—this vibration—so not only are you making this your point of attraction for those circumstances and experience, but this is also your lens through which you carry out those segments, so you act accordingly. This is how flow can be applied not only to those creative activities where you lose sense of time but to you living your life as well.

Segment intending has been invaluable to me in breaking free from a cycle I found myself in for so long. My past is laced with restricting and over-exercising during the week, and then come the weekend, I would drink too much, overeat, binge on occasion, and do it all over again. I hear a lot about similar cycles, even if it doesn't look exactly like this. When you are caught in a cycle such as this one, you are focused so much on the "not wanting" of the behavior: *I don't want to overeat, I don't want to drink too much, I don't want to binge.* For me, this focus and these thoughts kept me in a place of fear and anxiety. Although this was subconscious at the time, the weekend would roll around, and I would engage in the exact behaviors I was trying to shed in order to quell the negative emotions I was creating. It was one big feedback loop: a self-fulfilling prophecy.

Dieting, restriction, food rules, and a lack of self-love feed into the cycle. I noticed that when I started to focus on the *positive* emotions I wanted to feel, my choices, actions, and behaviors would unfold from that place, knowing that to stay aligned with this vision was something I had complete control over. Feeling so out of control had previously caused me to paint myself as a victim, leading to more disempowerment and even more anxiety.

In hindsight, I can recognize my ego through all of it. I realized that if I wanted things to change, it was not about the alcohol, the food, or how much exercise I engaged in to undo the damage. I had to change the way I thought about myself. My habitual thought patterns of guilt and shame were only causing more harm than good, keeping me stuck in the negative cycle. Making small mindset shifts to forgiveness first, and eventually peace and love, was when I could break free. My intentions made me more conscious, allowing me to connect to something deeper. Most importantly, I simultaneously learned to love myself.

As I have stated before, self-love must come first. A lack of self-love is directly proportionate to the disconnect between you and your inner being or intuition. It bears repeating: Your intuition only knows love; it has nothing but love for who "you" are. As Marianne Williamson describes in her book *A Return to Love*, "love is the intuitive knowledge of our hearts," and it is what we are all born with.[71]

When you allow your ego to take over, that is when you get the discrepancy of feeling at peace. It is important to remember that your ego does not like love. It wants to keep you separate from your intuition. If you are at peace and not alert and anxious, that is when danger catches you off guard. But this isn't the way our world works anymore. Every time your ego comes around with negative self-talk, you can say "Thank you, ego, for trying to keep me safe, but I am fine. You are free to go." Self-love is your authentic state of being, so it is time to take back your power.

journal:

> Now might be a good time to journal and write down everything you love about yourself. This exercise might be easier for some than for others, but everyone is capable of it. If a negative self-talk thought pops up, notice it, release it, and repeat one of the things you wrote down in your mind. It is going to take practice and it is going to take compassion.

Compassion is key. As a former perfectionist, the way I felt about myself was always connected to my achievements—those shiny pennies I would pick up, pat myself on the back, and feel good about myself for a little while. Yet it was fleeting and never felt sustainable because as humans, we are always looking for the next best thing or the next gold star to get. Instead, when you are more connected to your intuition, an inner love, and a deep sense of knowing how amazing you are, that is when feeling good becomes more consistent. It is innately rooted. It is also recognizing that there is no perfect, that as humans we will make mistakes, do things that don't serve us or others, and that is natural. Self-love does not come from only doing things "right"; it comes from loving yourself despite the "humanness" and occasionally making mistakes.

Katherine* approached me about health coaching for a couple of different reasons. Primarily, she wanted to find more balance with her eating, exercise, and mindset around wellness in general. She had always considered herself a healthy person: she enjoyed being active (is even a certified fitness instructor), loved to cook, and was interested in nutrition. She never thought of herself as a "dieter," per se, but realized that she basically had a dieting mindset. Her relationship with food was one that came with a lot of baggage, guilt, and stress. She had even found herself counting calories again in order to provide her eating with more structure, but that only made her scared to eat certain foods. She kept looking outside herself for answers, turning to what others in the wellness world were eating, projecting their lifestyles onto her own experience, which resulted in comparison. In her words, she wanted to get back to reality, to figure out her truth, not what anyone else thought was "healthy."

Throughout our sessions, she would have many "aha moments" that made her think her issues were primarily mental. She would release the stress, slow down, let go of the rules she had around food and exercise, adopt a more positive mindset, and embrace more pleasure in what she was eating. When she did, she would notice positive shifts. Her body would feel more balanced because she would have "let go" of all that pressure she was putting on herself. Although she refrained from weighing herself, she did confess during one of our conversations that she had lost a few pounds. She even made the connection between her previous mindset and digestive distress: While her diet didn't really change, her symptoms improved when she let go the fear and stress around food.

When I asked what her vision for better health entailed, she replied that she wanted peace. She wanted to feel confident that she was able to take care of herself no matter the situation she was in; that she could stop with the worrying, depriving, and restricting.

What I heard is that she wanted to increase her intuition and trust for herself.

In our work together, Katherine had many breakthroughs. First of all, she realized that all of the stories and thoughts she was telling herself about food and exercise were not only keeping her locked in this place of fear and anxiety, but also that the majority of what she was telling herself about her health wasn't even true. Her goal evolved: figure out her truth. She didn't want to look outside herself for answers. She wanted to get in tune to her body, her needs, not what others were doing or saying was right.

We discussed numerous mindset shifts, strategies, and action steps to keep her aligned with her vision.

In order to develop her self-trust, a big one at the beginning was to unfollow people on Instagram whom she felt weren't serving her anymore. She then learned to ask questions. For example, instead of waking up and telling herself she "had to" work out, she would ask, "What would feel best in my body today?" and do a form of movement (or no movement at all) that felt good.

She practiced being more present in order to clear the noise and clutter in her mind that was taking up headspace and energy. She did some journaling and daily affirmations to tap into the power of belief. She realized that when she "tried" too hard, things backfired, so she started to let go a little bit—less "efforting" while releasing the pressure she was putting on herself.

We talked through some things with food and exercise, and focused on those behaviors that were working *for* her rather than against her to stay focused on the positive and help find her truths. She started to look at her health habits through the lens of self-care rather than control. For example, knowing that when she ate a bigger breakfast and lunch, and a smaller dinner, this habit best served her energy and sleep. She wasn't depriving herself by eating a smaller dinner; that's just what made her feel best.

She dropped the word "should" from her vocabulary.

She released the rules and stopped weighing herself, and as a result, established new thoughts and beliefs. Basically, she had to learn to trust herself again after spending so much time in her former state of mind where that trust was repeatedly broken. This doesn't mean there weren't setbacks, especially when her ego resurfaced, but she navigated it beautifully, maintaining the notion that her mind was a key player in the process.

Something especially clicked with regard to calorie counting. She realized she was majorly overcomplicating food and nutrition. If she simplified, got back to basics, and ate more real, natural foods, she didn't have to count calories (which was only a form of control). Food didn't need to be moralized at all. She realized that for the time being, her body was asking for more plants, but this time, she didn't attach a label to it. She didn't need to denounce herself as a vegan or vegetarian to slide to a certain end of a spectrum to organize her eating. She simply made a point to eat more plants because that is what her body was asking for. This went against what she had previously been doing, as outside sources were emphasizing animal protein, but when she took a step back, she realized this path wasn't working for her. She almost immediately felt more intuitively balanced. She let go of the labels and approached each individual meal to figure out what foods would serve her best in the moment.

We worked on unblocking long-held beliefs and shedding old stories. She kept coming back to the thought that she was never doing enough. Using self-inquiry, she learned she was doing a lot—for her health and herself. Once she realized that, she felt more assured and peaceful about her daily habits and behaviors.

The biggest shift of all was that she started to approach this journey from a place of self-love rather than restriction. She felt lighter and more confident to navigate any situation, whether she was home or on the road traveling. Her journey may continue to ebb and flow, but her heightened sense of trust and alignment was her new foundation, and she could come back to it at any time. If she ever strayed from it, her body and emotions would tell her that much. Through conscious choice and intention, she could choose the thoughts that led to the feelings she wanted to feel: happy, light, and in the flow.

Toward the end of our work together, she sent me the following message:

> I continue to feel amazing! I just got back from a week-long trip in L.A. that I extended into a mini vacation with my husband, in which we ate out for almost every meal, ate sweet things, and things I would normally never touch, all without stress or stressing about exercising. I came back not having gained a pound, feeling just as healthy and like myself as when I left. You showed me my MIND was the missing piece and not some special diet or exercise routine. It's not even about the weight, it's just about feeling free and unstressed and excited about eating instead of fearful!

This work is about developing self-trust, leading with self-love, asking the right questions, increasing consciousness and intuition, letting go, shedding old stories, looking through a more positive lens, unblocking old beliefs and figuring out what is true, releasing the rules and external sources of control, and turning inward. The ultimate shift comes from focusing on your emotions first, and the way you want to feel, rather than on the physical conditions you think you need to have in place to be happy. Then when you can align your choices, habits, behavior, and energy with the feelings and not an attachment to a certain outcome, you will always know what is right and true for you.

journal:

I encourage you to uncover your truths. Here are some other important questions you could ask yourself: What is true for me? What do I like? What do I not like? What makes me feel good? What brings me joy? What doesn't? This could be related to food, exercise, your job, your pet, material possessions, or how you spend your time. Start jotting things down. Your body and intuition will tell you what is true. Yet turning inward doesn't mean you have to throw nutritional caution to the wind; you can still be a student in this sense. I often tell my clients that there are a lot of different dietary theories out there; fads and trends tend to cause confusion. A common thread, however, has always been to eat more real food, and vegetables are good for you. Within those parameters, where can you add in, release the rules and restrictions, and practice more peace in mindful eating?

Then use your emotions and inner compass as a guide to keep you aligned. Without judgement for your past, use the experiences you have had thus far to provide information and reflection for answers. If you write something down that does not feel true, your body and intuition will tell you. If you write down "I love kale" because your mind tells you that you should love kale, but you feel a sensation in your chest or gut that doesn't feel like loving kale, notice that and perhaps scratch it out. Truth feels like alignment. Alignment feels like a deep *knowing*.

Bring this exercise to those parts of your life that might feel out of balance. Are there any aspects of your career, creativity, relationships, or spirituality where you are not fully speaking or living your truth? Where you feel stuck and "flow-less"? Even if you can't make any sweeping changes overnight, where can you incorporate more flow to offset any feelings of imbalance?

When I was working a corporate job in my mid-twenties, I felt very unfulfilled. This is when I started my first healthy-living blog, on which I would document recipes and workouts. I absolutely loved it, and would work on it during those "fringe hours" of the early mornings and evenings. Although I didn't consciously realize it at the time, this was the first time I experienced flow— being so *joyfully* immersed in something that I lost track of time. The juxtaposition wasn't lost on me. To feel so happy and aligned doing one thing, and then having to spend nine or ten hours doing something I did not enjoy, brought the desire to make a change "front and center." Blogging built the springboard for how I wanted to feel *most* of the time, not just for a couple of hours a day. To create a life I loved meant not just having a creative hobby (although that is how it started) but also believing I *deserved* alignment and fulfillment in my career, creativity, and relationships. When you understand what alignment feels like for you, you can apply it to any area of your life. When I shifted from seeking fulfillment from the physical aspects of my "self" (the number on the scale, body image), to asking what would make my heart happy, that is when all of the issues around food and weight started to fall away.

That is not to say my path from that point has been one of pure alignment. There have been changes, challenges, and roadblocks along the way. From major life events, like the death of loved ones, business failures, and the COVID-19 pandemic, to feeling stuck in a rut without a reason why. It is during these times when my unhealthy habits and programming around food and weight can resurface to distract me; to overshadow the deeper, more uncomfortable emotions from which my mind wants to protect me. Having done so much work on myself, I always understand what is taking place, and I can use consciousness to "disrupt the drift," give myself permission to feel the feelings, surrender what I can't control, count colors to focus on the good and gratitude, find something that gets be back in the flow, and stay the course to a better, more balanced state. It is a journey, process, and practice; our biggest work as a human being, but also the greatest gift.

So I ask: What if we made our wellness about an inward experience instead of an outward one? Our journey toward better health would be about our heart and soul rather than weight and image. In the turning inward, our health becomes more about the love and alignment of feeling good, and not about our insecurities or parts of ourselves we felt needed fixing. From the foundation of feeling good is where we choose. Our ability to tap into intrinsic motivation would strengthen. We wouldn't need an app or Instagram influencer to inspire our self-care. We wouldn't allow comparison to influence feelings of "not enough." We wouldn't fall victim to our past, blame our genes, or feel stuck in the way things are because that is how they have been, even though it doesn't align with how we want them to be. We would navigate our days from already feeling enough. We would have the ability to meet the moment with confidence and compassion. With the ability to be more conscious and present, you empower yourself to follow the unfolding of your moments with more clarity and intention. In these moments, you see more beauty in yourself and daily life by counting the colors around you, feeling grateful for what is already there, and excited for all that is to come. This does not mean that health-supportive practices, such as nutrition and exercise, fall by the wayside; instead, they become ingrained in who you are because you care. That is what self-care is all about.

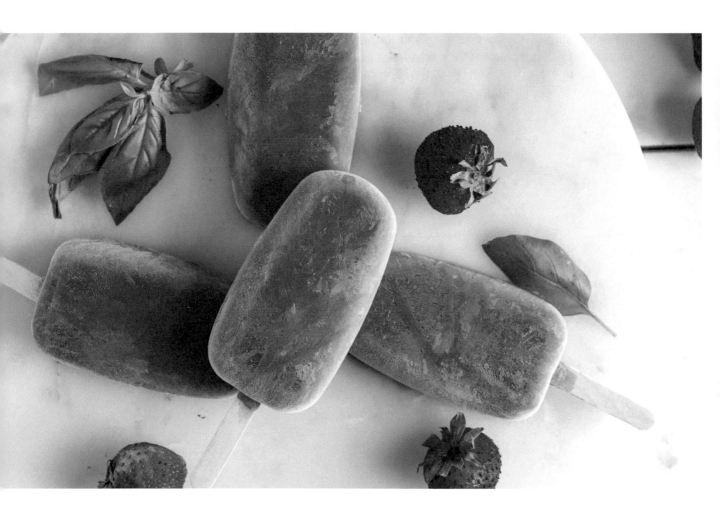

epilogue

*W*hat started out as a simple nutritional mantra has become a portal to consciousness. Through mindfulness for the present moment, you can access your true self. You can strip away the layers of conditioning, habit, and stories that no longer serve you. It takes awareness, work, and patience, but ironically, it can be as simple as *feeling* present. The Counting Colors philosophy offers you a tool to more easily do so. To "wake up" to yourself, and tap in to those emotions you have been wanting to feel all along when you might have been looking outside of yourself for the answers.

Before we part ways, it is important to bring up a couple of realizations I have had about my own mindfulness since starting this book. First, the fact that "being present" has almost become cliché in the wellness world has encouraged me to explore its true meaning *for me*, using the power of questions to peel back the layers and shed beliefs to become a more peaceful version of myself, and I encourage you to do the same. We all long to feel more present, yet it is an abstract concept, one that can be difficult to grasp. This is because you cannot "think" your way to the present moment. Not only can the mind not easily conceive of it, but it is the job of the mind to take you out of it. Rather, it is something that is felt and experienced through the five senses of the body, sight being an initial access switch and anchor.

This led me to ask: Why do I want to feel more present? It offers the promise of peace and freedom—there is a savoring of joy that can be felt when fully present, but the present moment is always fleeting. This peace and freedom then feel like an illusion, always beyond my grasp; or if felt, it is gone as quickly as it came. As soon as I feel as if I have dropped in, the next thought takes me out. Perhaps it is a thought analyzing the experience, creating a story around it, or it isn't related to the experience at all, but rather a thought tethered to the past or future. This natural tendency of the mind is compounded by the amount of distraction that surrounds us on a daily basis. I believe our society at large is constantly distracted; if it is not our thoughts that take us out of the present moment, it is the ding of our phones, the emails and media, comparison to other people's lives, wrapped in a layer of the stories and meaning we attach to these things. This creates a drift down a rabbit hole of more swirling stories and thoughts, and we are no longer in the now. This begs the question: What purpose does distraction serve?

It is a numbing agent for the present moment. As much as we desire more presence in our lives, "being present" can often feel uncomfortable, seemingly disproving the freedom and peace theory. But why? Why has a research study shown that people would rather shock themselves than be alone with their thoughts? And therein lies the paradox. I have seen this in myself when I have succumbed to distraction. I want so badly to feel more present—both consciously and subconsciously—when I find myself constantly trying to run from the moment. Without the outside distraction, what is buried deep inside can surface. Shame, guilt, trauma, fear, and any other uncomfortable emotions that coincide are heavy burdens to bear. We therefore distract and numb and place our attention on those parts of ourselves that give us a modicum of control, our physical body being one of them. But as uncomfortable as they can be, they are emotions after all. We can all survive emotions. Research shows the lifespan of emotions is ninety seconds; it is our mind, attachment to them, and stories around them that elongates the hold they have over us.

Is it therefore a matter of getting more comfortable in the discomfort, or do I simply need to shift my perspective in the present moment to find more inner peace? Knowing that in the true present moment there is only what *is*—the colors, sights, sounds—and my attention to what is, rather than that which may be causing the discomfort in the first place. Learning to pay attention to your attention is mindfulness, the moment-to-moment awareness, and the ticket to ultimate freedom and peace.

The answers for you can only be found in your own self-exploration, and I am hoping this book and its teachings offer a springboard to connect to your "self" as it has for me. When you become more conscious, you cannot go back to the way you were before. You cannot unsee what you have seen. It is like an ocular illusion—your eyes initially strain and struggle to see the hidden image sitting right on the surface. Once you catch a glimpse, seeing it again becomes much more seamless, and you wonder how you missed it in the first place. Becoming more conscious provides you with a new level of awareness that is always with you; it starts out as a whisper, but as you continue to practice, it only grows to become a more significant aspect of the way your mind works. You might not be able to completely rid yourself of old mental habits and programming, but becoming more conscious of them, you gain a sense of empowerment to select another thought, make another choice. The awareness provides you the ability to write a new story, rather than staying stuck in one that no longer serves your highest self.

Looking back on my story, I not only feel compassion for my past relationship with food and my body but also gratitude, as it sparked this evolution to consciousness. In those moments when I notice old fears and patterns of thought creep back in (because they do, especially during times of stress or when I feel out of control in other aspects of life), I can use the Counting Colors philosophy to get back to a better feeling place. True freedom cannot be found in the number on the scale, just as it cannot be found in other circumstances outside of yourself that only result in ephemeral feelings of "happiness." As soon as we pick up a shiny penny, we are looking for the next one. True freedom is found through a deeper connection to your intuition and the knowing you can feel the freedom *first*, here and now.

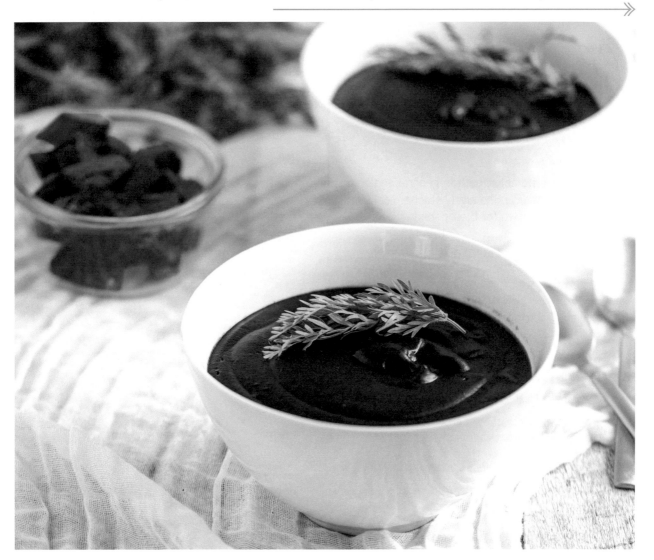

recipes

blue-berry
VANILLA SMOOTHIE

Makes 2 servings

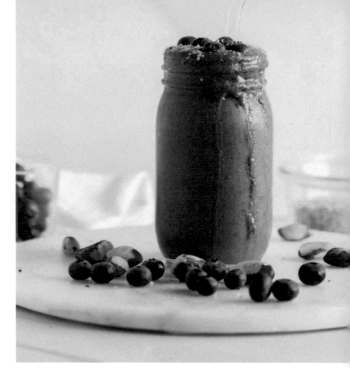

Blue is my favorite color, both in general and in nutrition. Anthocyanins are phytochemicals found in plants known for their potent antioxidant properties. They contribute the beautiful blue and purple hues found in plant-based foods. Blueberries, blackberries, and purple cabbage are prime examples, and all three are used in this smoothie recipe to provide you that powerful nutritional punch.

ingredients

- 1½–2 cups dairy-free milk of choice (or filtered water)
- ½ cup frozen blueberries
- ½ cup frozen blackberries
- ⅓–½ frozen banana
- 1½ cups chopped raw purple cabbage (see note)
- 1 tablespoon nut or seed butter (such as almond or cashew)
- 1 tablespoon chia seeds or psyllium husk
- 1 scoop vanilla protein powder

directions

1. In a high-speed blender, combine the dairy-free milk, frozen blueberries, frozen blackberries, frozen banana, purple cabbage, nut butter, chia seeds or psyllium husk, and vanilla protein powder.
2. Blend on high for 1 to 2 minutes until a smooth and creamy consistency is reached. (If you are using a Vitamix, use the tamper as you need to get everything going.)
3. Pour the smoothie into two glasses and serve.

notes

» *You can use fresh blueberries, but this will affect the consistency of the smoothie.*

» *If you experience digestive issues with raw vegetables, steam your cabbage before using or freezing it.*

strawberry
MACA GREEN SMOOTHIE

Makes 2 servings

Thanks to the use of spinach or kale, green is the color that shines through in this smoothie. This recipe follows a blood sugar balancing format, and the frozen cauliflower adds to the base without adding to the sugar. Strawberries pair well with maca powder, which is an adaptogen known to support hormonal balance, increase energy, and enhance mood and memory.

ingredients

- 1½–2 cups dairy-free milk of choice (or filtered water)
- ½ cup frozen strawberries
- ½ cup frozen cauliflower rice or florets
- ⅓–½ frozen banana
- 2 cups fresh spinach or kale (or leafy greens of choice)
- 1 tablespoon nut or seed butter (such as almond or cashew)
- 1 tablespoon chia seeds or psyllium husk
- 1 scoop vanilla protein powder
- 1 teaspoon maca powder

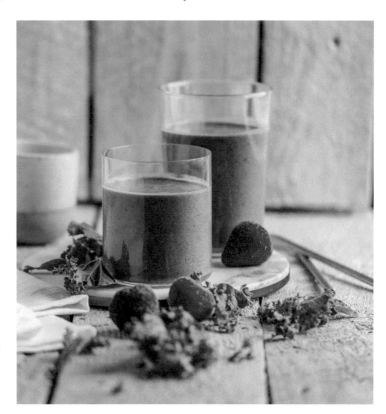

directions

1. In a high-speed blender, combine the dairy-free milk, frozen strawberries, frozen cauliflower, frozen banana, spinach or kale, nut butter, chia seeds or psyllium husk, vanilla protein powder, and maca powder.

2. Blend on high for 1 to 2 minutes until a smooth and creamy consistency is reached. (If you are using a Vitamix, use the tamper as you need to get everything going.)

3. Pour the smoothie into two glasses and serve.

notes

» *You can use fresh strawberries or banana, but this will affect the consistency of the smoothie.*

» *If you experience digestive issues with raw vegetables, steam your cauliflower before using or freezing it.*

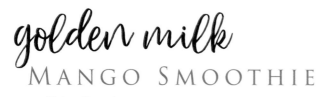

golden milk
MANGO SMOOTHIE

Makes 2 servings
Recipe by Kate Stephenson

This smoothie is creamy, refreshing, sweet, and tart all at the same time. Turmeric contributes its golden color, but you can't taste it. This drink is especially great if you need some detox support, as both the grapefruit and the turmeric naturally support your detoxification pathways.

ingredients

- 1 cup dairy-free milk of choice (or filtered water)
- 1 cup frozen mango
- ½ cup frozen cauliflower rice
- ½ fresh or frozen banana (use frozen for a creamier consistency)
- Juice from ½ grapefruit (equals about ¼ cup)
- 1 tablespoon hemp hearts
- ¼ teaspoon grated fresh ginger
- A pinch of ground turmeric (equals about ⅛ teaspoon)

directions

1. In a high-speed blender, combine the dairy-free milk, mango, cauliflower rice, banana, grapefruit juice, hemp hearts, ginger, and turmeric.
2. Blend on high for 1 to 2 minutes until smooth and creamy. (If you are using a Vitamix, use the tamper as you need to get everything going.)
3. Pour the smoothie into two glasses and serve.

notes

» *Most grocery stores have bags of pre-riced cauliflower rice. Some brands are already frozen, which makes keeping cauliflower rice on hand pretty easy. I buy a bag from the produce section at Whole Foods and throw it into my freezer as soon as I get home.*

» *To make this smoothie lower in sugar, substitute an extra ½ cup of cauliflower rice for the frozen banana.*

» *To juice your grapefruit, cut it in half, pierce the inner flesh with a fork to start releasing the juices, and then squeeze.*

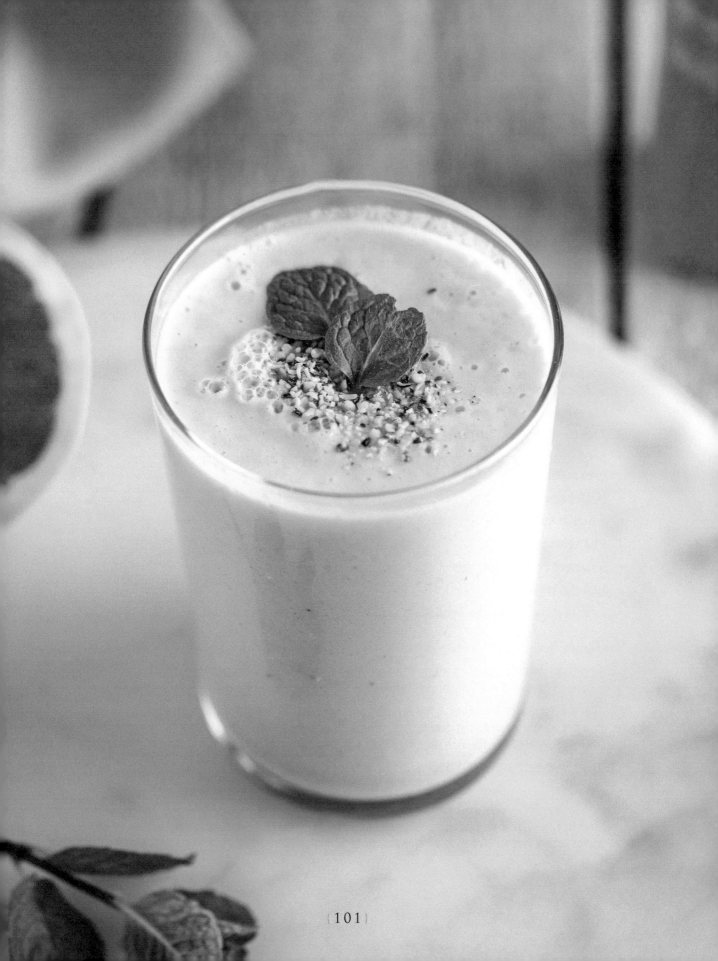

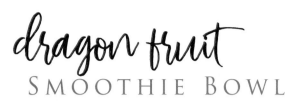

dragon fruit
SMOOTHIE BOWL

Makes 1 serving
Recipe by Kate Stephenson

When it comes to a colorful smoothie bowl, there is nothing prettier than Pitaya. In its full form, the fruit has a pink and spiky exterior, hence its nickname: dragon fruit. On the inside, you will find either white or red flesh speckled with seeds. It's the latter that is harvested and put into little packs that makes this nutrient-dense smoothie bowl possible. The lemon and ginger provide a refreshing flavor, while the chia seeds, spinach, and cauliflower add even more plant-based nutrition. This smoothie bowl makes counting colors easy! Add your favorite toppings to round out the recipe.

ingredients

- ½ cup dairy-free milk of choice
  (or filtered water or coconut water)
- 1 large handful fresh spinach
- 1 cup frozen strawberries (or raspberries)
- 1 (3.5-ounce) Dragon Fruit/Pitaya Pack, roughly chopped into chunks (or ½ cup of Dragon Fruit Cubes (such as Pitaya brand)
- ⅓ cup frozen cauliflower rice
- ½ fresh or frozen banana
- 2 teaspoons chia seeds
- ½ teaspoon freshly grated ginger
- Juice of ½ lemon
- Toppings of choice (examples: hemp hearts, nuts, berries, bananas, shredded coconut, granola, bee pollen)

directions

1. In a high-speed blender combine the dairy-free milk, fresh spinach, frozen strawberries, chopped Dragon Fruit/Pitaya, cauliflower rice, banana, chia seeds, ginger, and lemon juice.

2. Blend on high for 2 minutes until smooth and creamy. (If you are using a Vitamix, use the tamper as you need to get everything going.) The mixture will be thick! You might need to stop the blender halfway through and give the mixture a stir with a spatula.

3. Transfer the smoothie to a bowl and add toppings.

notes

» *To reduce the sugar content in this recipe, look for unsweetened Dragon Fruit/Pitaya packs. You can also substitute an extra ⅓ cup of frozen cauliflower rice for the banana, but it may affect the consistency.*

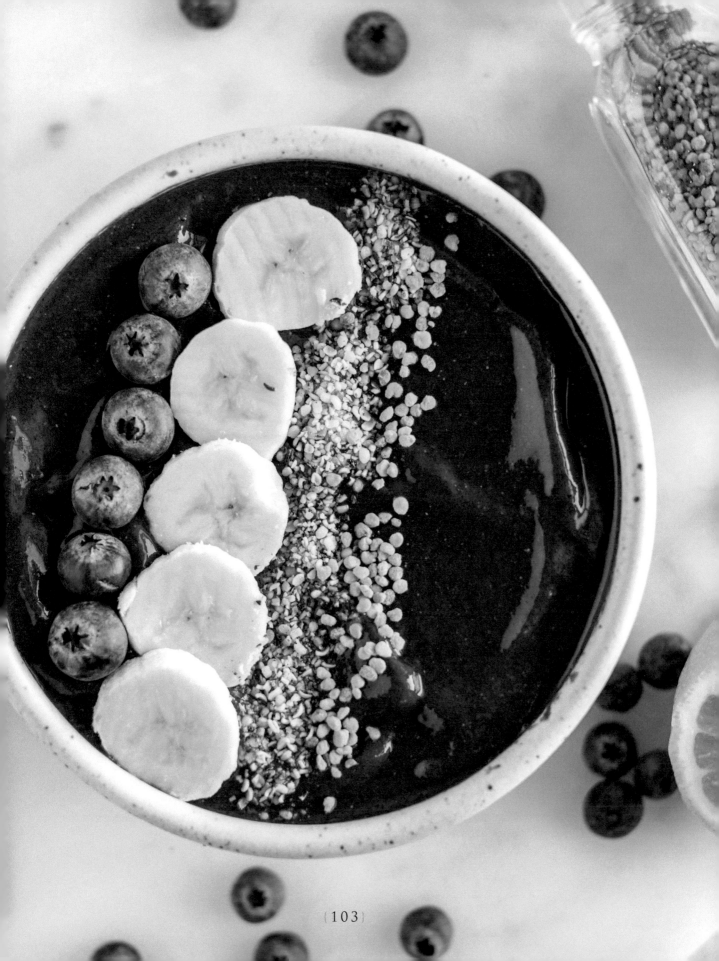

blue chia
PUDDING PARFAITS

Makes 2 servings

Who knew something so beautiful could pack such a powerful nutritional punch? The blue hue of this chia pudding parfait is pure magic. The blue algae spirulina comes in a couple of different forms, and the powder extract not only lends its pigment but also its anti-inflammatory and antioxidant effects. Paired with chia seeds, this breakfast option is full of superfoods.

ingredients

- 1 cup dairy-free milk of choice (such as almond or coconut)
- 1 teaspoon blue spirulina powder
- 1 teaspoon vanilla extract
- 1 tablespoon maple syrup (optional)
- ¼ cup chia seeds
- ½ cup coconut yogurt, divided (or yogurt of choice)
- Toppings: fresh berries, unsweetened shredded coconut

directions

1. In a small bowl or mason jar, combine the dairy-free milk, blue spirulina powder, vanilla extract, and maple syrup if using. Whisk until blended.

2. Add the chia seeds and stir vigorously until incorporated into the wet mixture. Continue to stir occasionally for 5 to 10 minutes to prevent the chia mixture from clumping.

3. Transfer the chia pudding to the refrigerator for at least one hour or ideally overnight to set. Once set, layer the chia pudding with coconut yogurt. Add toppings if desired.

notes

» *Full-fat coconut milk will make the chia pudding creamier.*

» *If you want to add more protein to this recipe, stir in 1 tablespoon of collagen with the wet ingredients; it's tasteless, so it will not affect the flavor.*

» *Blue spirulina is different from green spirulina due to the pigment phycocyanin, which delivers its unique benefits. You can use green spirulina in this recipe, but the resulting color will be green and may affect the taste.*

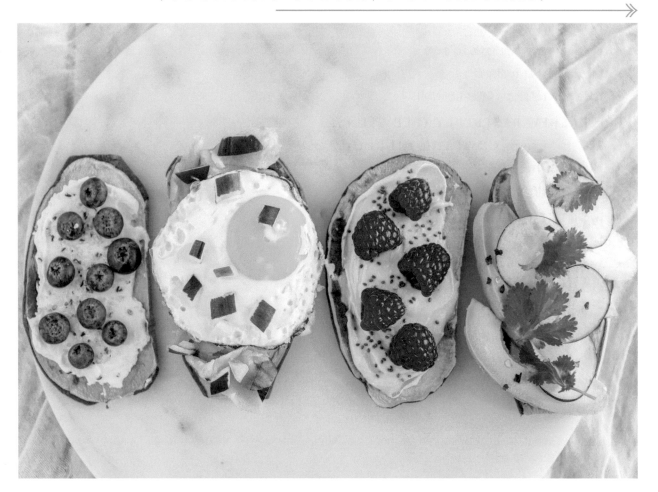

sweet potato toast
— 4 WAYS

Makes 2 to 3 servings (depending on the size of the sweet potato)

Sweet potato makes for a colorful swap for traditional toast. Not only does it make a great base for your favorite toppings, but it is also a good source of fiber, vitamins A and C, manganese, and potassium. Add extra color to your sweet potato toast by using the toppings below, or choose your own.

ingredients

- 1 medium sweet potato
- Cooking spray or cooking oil (see note)
- Sea salt and black pepper to taste
- Toppings of choice (see variations)

FOR AVOCADO (PER SLICE):

- ½ avocado, thinly sliced (or substitute with 2 tablespoons guacamole)

continued

- 1 small radish, thinly sliced
- 1 tablespoon roughly chopped cilantro
- Juice from ¼ lime (optional)
- ½ teaspoon red pepper flakes (optional)

FOR CASHEW RASPBERRY (PER SLICE):

- 2 tablespoons creamy cashew butter (or nut butter of choice)
- ¼ cup fresh raspberries
- ½ teaspoon chia seeds (optional)

FOR SMOKED SALMON (PER SLICE):

- 1–2 thin slices smoked salmon
- 1 egg, sunny-side up or poached (optional)
- 1 tablespoon red onion, thinly sliced

FOR COCONUT BLUEBERRY (PER SLICE):

- 2 tablespoons coconut yogurt (or yogurt of choice)
- ¼ cup fresh blueberries
- ½ teaspoon hemp seeds (optional)

directions

1. Cut sweet potato lengthwise into ¼-inch-thick slices. Spray each slice with cooking spray or thinly coat with oil.

2. Turn toaster on medium-high and toast 2 or 3 times until the sweet potato is fork tender. If using the oven, preheat the oven to 400° F. Lay the sweet potato toasts flat on a baking sheet, and bake for 15 to 20 minutes until fork tender, turning them over about halfway through cooking. You can also place them directly onto the oven rack.

3. Allow the sweet potato slices to slightly cool (about 5 to 10 minutes) before adding toppings.

notes

» *For the cooking spray, I suggest an avocado-oil-based cooking spray like Primal Kitchen or Chosen Foods brands. You can also coat the pan with 1 teaspoon of cooking oil per slice (avocado oil, olive oil, or melted coconut oil).*

» *The length of cooking time will depend on your toaster or oven. Aim for slightly crispy edges with a fork-tender center.*

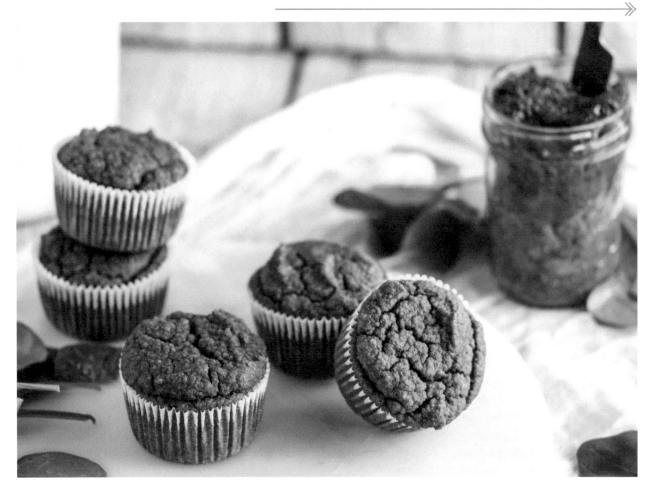

green banana muffins
WITH STRAWBERRY CHIA JAM

Makes 10 to 12 muffins

Whether you want to sneak in an extra vegetable for yourself or a loved one, these green banana muffins will do the trick. You can enjoy the nutrition of spinach without having to taste it. Enjoy a muffin with vibrant strawberry chia jam for extra color, plant-based protein, healthy fat, and flavor.

ingredients

FOR THE MUFFINS:

- 1½ cups almond flour
- ¼ cup coconut flour
- ¼ cup tapioca starch
- 1 teaspoon baking powder
- 1 teaspoon cinnamon

continued

- ½ teaspoon baking soda
- ¼ teaspoon sea salt
- ½ cup dairy-free milk of choice
- 2 very ripe bananas
- 2 eggs
- 4 loosely packed cups fresh spinach
- 2 tablespoons maple syrup or honey
- 1 teaspoon vanilla extract

FOR THE STRAWBERRY CHIA JAM:

- 1 cup frozen strawberries
- 1 teaspoon vanilla extract
- 2 tablespoons chia seeds

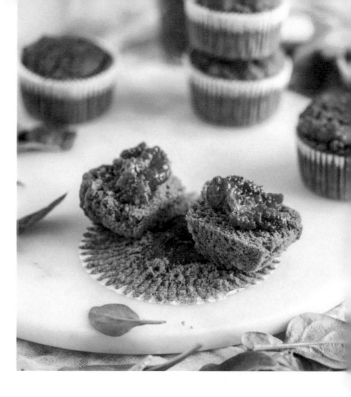

directions

1. To make the muffins: Preheat the oven to 350° F. Line a muffin tin with liners.

2. In a large mixing bowl, combine the almond flour, coconut flour, tapioca starch, baking powder, cinnamon, baking soda, and sea salt. Stir to blend, breaking up any clumps with a spoon or spatula.

2. In a high-speed blender, combine the dairy-free milk, bananas, eggs, spinach, maple syrup or honey, and vanilla extract. Process on low speed, gradually increasing the speed to high until blended and creamy (about 45 seconds). You can also use a food processor for this step, but the consistency might not be as creamy.

3. Pour the wet ingredients into the mixing bowl with the flour mixture. Whisk until a batter is formed.

4. Pour the batter into the muffin tin, filling each liner about three-fourths of the way to the top. Bake 23 to 25 minutes, or until a toothpick inserted in the center comes out clean. Allow the muffins to completely cool in the muffin tin, at least 1 hour.

5. To make the strawberry chia jam: Place the frozen strawberries in a small saucepan over medium heat. Cook for 5 to 6 minutes until the strawberries start to thaw and release their juices, stirring occasionally. As the strawberries continue to thaw and soften, continue to cook and stir, mashing them with the back of a wooden spoon until a jam-like consistency is reached, about 5 more minutes. Add the vanilla extract and chia seeds. Stir to combine, and then remove the saucepan from heat. Continue to stir occasionally while the chia seeds gel, at least 10 minutes.

6. When ready to serve, spoon the strawberry chia jam on top of a muffin or muffin halves. Serve warm.

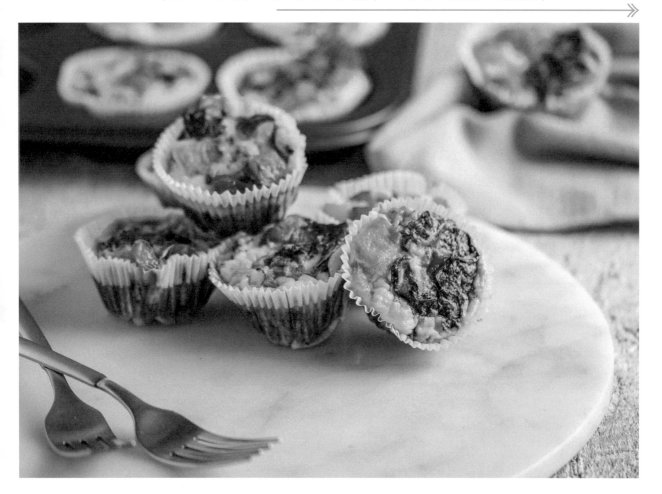

colorful egg
MUFFINS

Makes 10 to 12 muffins

In addition to the colorful vegetables found inside, these egg muffins come with an extra benefit: batch cooking! Make them once, and have a quick breakfast or snack to grab on the go all week. They even freeze well. While I offer a recipe here, know that these egg muffins are very versatile.

ingredients

- 2 tablespoons olive oil or avocado oil for cooking
- ½ red bell pepper, cored, seeded, and diced
- ½ green bell pepper, cored, seeded, and diced
- ½ yellow bell pepper, cored, seeded, and diced
- 2 cups chopped curly kale
- 8 eggs, beaten

continued

- ½ teaspoon garlic powder
- ½ teaspoon onion powder
- ¼ cup crumbled goat cheese or feta cheese (optional)
- Sea salt and black pepper to taste

directions

1. Preheat the oven to 375° F. Line a muffin tin with liners.

2. Heat oil in a medium skillet over medium heat. Add the diced bell peppers and a sprinkle of sea salt and black pepper, and cook until softened and the bell pepper has brightened in color, about 7 to 10 minutes. Add the chopped kale and cook an additional 2 minutes, stirring frequently until the kale is wilted.

3. In a large bowl, combine the beaten eggs, garlic powder, onion powder, cheese (if using), cooked bell peppers and kale, and another dash of sea salt and black pepper. Stir until all ingredients are blended.

4. Spoon the mixture evenly between the muffin liners, filling each one about two-thirds full. Cook 18 to 20 minutes until set. Allow the egg muffins to cool for at least 15 to 20 minutes in the muffin tin. Enjoy warm, or allow them to cool completely at room temperature, about 1 hour.

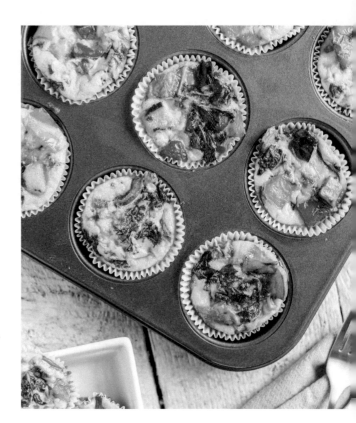

notes

» *You can use spinach instead of kale.*

» *The above recipe offers an example, but any cooked or roasted vegetable works! Think broccoli, chopped asparagus, mushrooms, or other sauteed greens.*

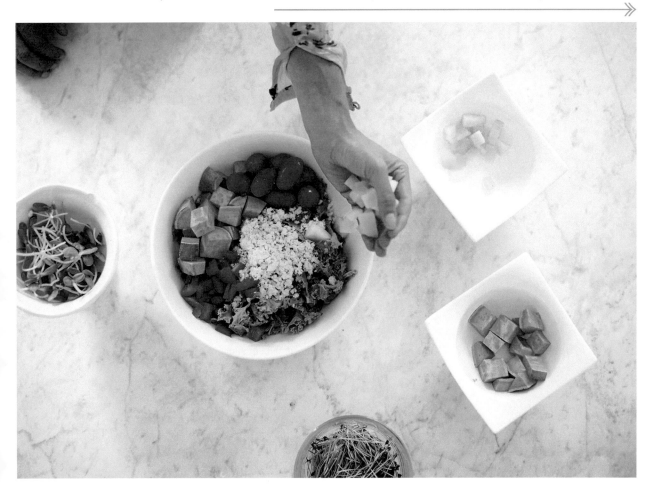

create on canvas
BUDDHA BOWL

Serves 1

One of my favorite lunches or dinners (especially toward the end of the week) is to throw together a big, colorful Buddha bowl salad made up of a variety of vegetables and/or fruits, high-quality protein, and healthy fat. This is a good opportunity to use up any leftovers from the work week. Bring everything together with your dressing of choice. There is no "recipe," per se, just a formula, and the goal is to incorporate as many colors (nutrients) as you can.

ingredient suggestions

FOR THE BASE:

- Spinach
- Kale
- Mixed greens
- Microgreens

continued

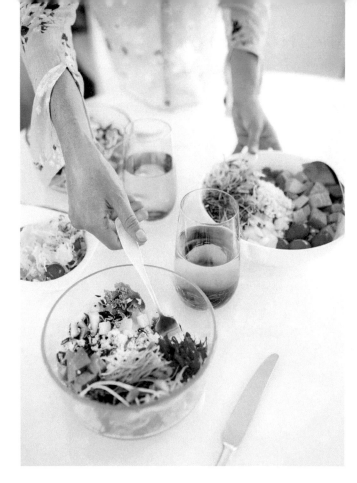

- Chopped romaine lettuce
- Shredded cabbage
- Zucchini noodles

FOR THE VEGETABLES/FRUITS:

- Brussels sprouts
- Asparagus
- Diced sweet potato
- Diced butternut squash
- Mushrooms
- Diced apple
- Berries
- Pomegranate seeds
- Sauerkraut
- Cucumber
- Zucchini or summer squash
- Roasted red peppers
- Broccoli (raw or roasted)
- Cauliflower florets (raw or roasted)
- Cauliflower rice (raw or roasted)
- Olives
- Avocado
- Grape tomatoes

FOR THE PROTEIN:

- Grilled or rotisserie chicken
- Create on Canvas Buddha Bowl (continued)
- Egg (hard-boiled or sunny-side up)
- Smoked salmon
- Pan-seared or baked fish (salmon, tuna, cod, etc.)
- Homemade chicken or tuna salad
- Sardines
- Grass-fed beef, bison, or turkey (burger patty or meatballs)
- All-natural, nitrate-free bacon
- Cooked shrimp

OTHER:

- Nuts or seeds for topping
- Hemp hearts
- Chia seeds
- Cheese (goat, feta, shredded cheese of choice) (omit for dairy-free)
- Cooked quinoa or rice
- Fresh herbs

DRESSING SUGGESTIONS

Simple Balsamic Vinaigrette:

- 2 tablespoons olive oil
- 2 tablespoons balsamic vinegar
- 1 teaspoon Dijon mustard
- ½ teaspoon honey (omit for sugar-free)
- Sea salt and black pepper to taste

Apple Cider Vinaigrette:

- ½ cup olive oil
- ¼ cup apple cider vinegar
- 1 tablespoon Dijon mustard
- Juice from ½ lemon
- Sea salt and black pepper to taste

Tahini-Turmeric Dressing:

- 1 tablespoon creamy tahini
- 1 tablespoon olive oil
- 1 teaspoon maple syrup (optional)
- ¼ teaspoon turmeric
- Dash of black pepper, sea salt to taste

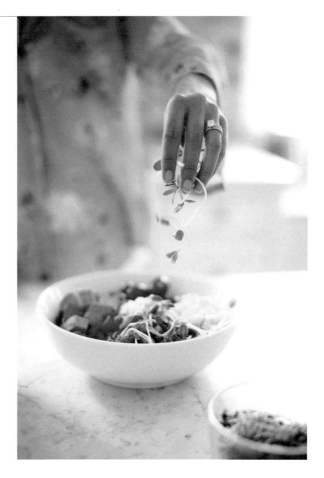

directions

1. In a mixing bowl, combine all desired Buddha bowl ingredients. Use a salad chopper or knife to prepare the ingredients.
2. To make the dressing: Combine the ingredients in a small bowl. Whisk until creamy.
3. Toss the Buddha bowl ingredients in the dressing of choice, and serve.

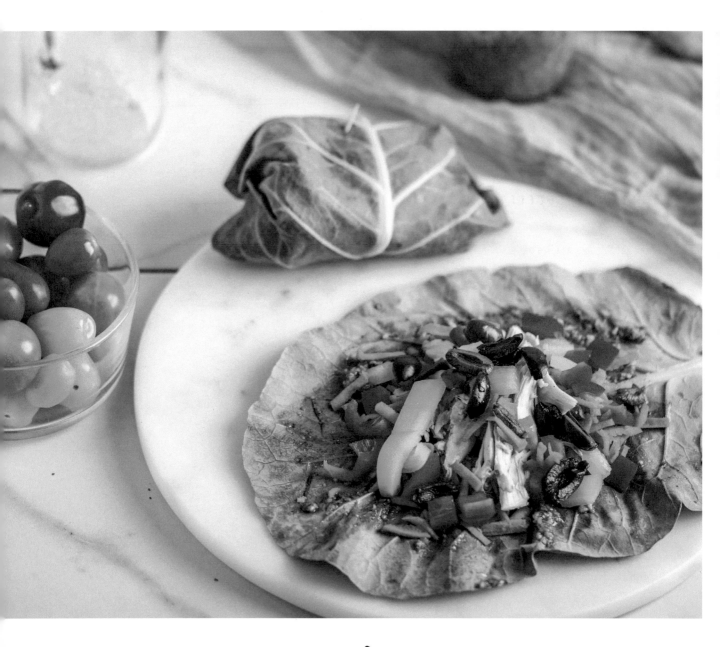

colorful collard wraps
WITH DAIRY-FREE PESTO

Makes 2 wraps

When I was exploring a gluten-free lifestyle, I needed a substitution for my go-to lunch wrap. Collard leaves offer a great option! Not only do they act as a tortilla substitute but you will also be eating a healthy leafy green over a processed food. In other words, a shift from a "brown" food to a more colorful food. Automatically get your greens in with the wrap itself, and incorporate other vegetables to count more colors. Find my ingredient suggestions below.

ingredients

FOR THE PESTO:

- 1 cup packed fresh basil
- 1 cup raw walnuts
- ½ cup olive oil (plus more if needed)
- 3 garlic cloves
- Juice from ½ lemon
- 2 teaspoons nutritional yeast (optional)

FOR THE COLLARD WRAPS:

- 2 large collard leaves
- ¼ cup dairy-free pesto
- 4 ounces chopped grilled chicken or rotisserie chicken (equals about 1 cup cooked) (omit for vegan)
- ½ avocado
- 1 large carrot, grated (equals about ⅓ cup)
- ¼ red bell pepper, small dice
- ¼ yellow bell pepper, small dice
- ¼ cup pitted, halved kalamata olives
- Brown mustard for dipping (optional)

directions

1. To make the pesto: In a food processor, combine the fresh basil, walnuts, olive oil, garlic, lemon juice, and nutritional yeast if using. Blend until creamy and ingredients are incorporated together, scraping down the sides of the food processor and pulsing as needed. If the pesto is too chunky, add more olive oil 1 tablespoon at a time while the food processor is going until the desired consistency is reached. Use on your collard wraps immediately, and store any leftover in an airtight container in the refrigerator for up to 1 week.

2. Prepare the collard leaves by using a sharp paring knife to remove the thick stem at the base of each collard leaf. Shave down the stem that runs along the leaf as much as you can, until the spine and leaf are even. You can blanch the leaf in simmering water for 30 seconds to make it more malleable for folding, otherwise lay the raw leaf flat on a cutting board or counter.

3. Add the ingredients. Spread on the pesto first, using about 2 tablespoons per leaf. Add chicken (if using), avocado, grated carrots, bell pepper, and olives. Fold each leaf as you would a tortilla: fold in the sides and then roll. Use a knife to slice each leaf in half or eat whole. Dip in brown mustard if desired.

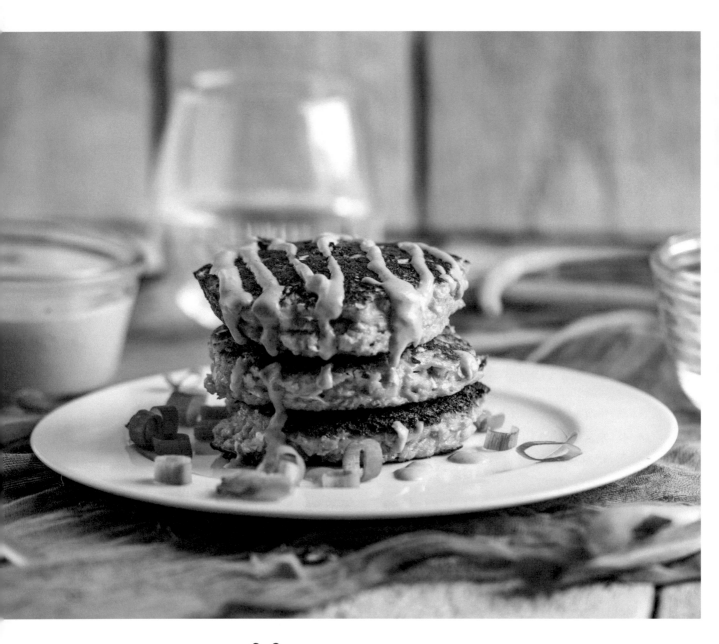

green cabbage patties
WITH SRIRACHA AIOLI

Makes 4 patties

When my husband and I were on our honeymoon, we had the most delicious Japanese pancake as an appetizer. This dish is made with cabbage and served with a dipping sauce. Upon returning home, I immediately tried to recreate it. I have evolved the recipe over the years, and this rendition has been the one that has stuck. Cabbage can be a bland food, but when you make these patties, there is nothing bland about them, especially when drizzled with the Sriracha aioli.

ingredients

FOR THE CABBAGE PANCAKES:

- 3 scallions
- 2 cups finely shredded green cabbage (from an 8-ounce box of pre-shredded cabbage or one small head of green cabbage) (see note)
- ¾ cup almond flour
- 1 teaspoon minced ginger
- 2 tablespoons coconut aminos
- 2 eggs, beaten
- 2 tablespoons avocado oil or coconut oil for cooking

FOR THE SRIRACHA AIOLI:

- ½ cup mayonnaise
- ½ cup ketchup
- 2 teaspoons sriracha (or hot sauce of choice)

directions

1. To make the cabbage pancakes: Thinly slice the scallions, separating the white ends from the green stems. Set the green slices aside.

2. In a large bowl, combine the scallion white ends, shredded green cabbage, almond flour, ginger, and coconut aminos. Stir to blend. Add the beaten egg and mix well until all ingredients are coated in the egg.

3. Heat the oil in a large skillet over medium heat. Use your hands to form patties of equal size, about 3 to 4 inches in diameter. Cook 4 to 5 minutes. Flip and cook an additional 4 to 5 more minutes. Remove from the heat and set aside.

4. To make the dipping sauce: In a medium bowl, combine the mayonnaise, ketchup, and Sriracha. Drizzle the aioli on top of each pancake or use as a dipping sauce. Garnish with the green scallion slices.

notes

» *If you have a food processor, I recommend using it. If you are using a whole head of cabbage, you can roughly chop it by hand first, and then finely shred it in a food processor. I typically use a box of pre-shredded cabbage, and I still pulse it in the food processor to get it more finely shredded.*

» *You can substitute tamari or soy sauce for the coconut aminos, but both substitutions will result in the recipe containing soy (tamari is gluten-free, whereas soy sauce typically is not).*

» *Purple cabbage won't work in this recipe, as it tends to be thicker than green cabbage.*

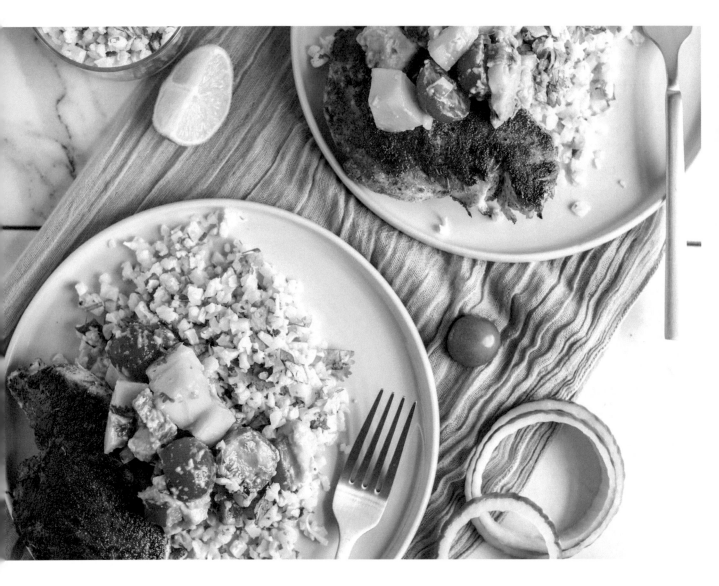

jerk chicken

WITH CILANTRO LIME CAULIFLOWER RICE

and mango salsa

Makes 4 servings

I love a tropical flavor profile. When you travel to an island culture, you will not only notice a lot of colorful foods, but they are also amazingly fresh, usually grown in a garden right around the corner from the restaurant. This recipe brings a taste of the islands right into your kitchen.

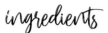
ingredients

FOR THE CHICKEN:

- 2 teaspoons garlic powder
- 2 teaspoons onion powder
- 1 teaspoon cayenne pepper
- 1 teaspoons sea salt
- 1 teaspoon ground black pepper
- 1 teaspoon coconut sugar
- ½ teaspoon dried thyme
- ½ teaspoon paprika
- ½ teaspoon cumin
- ½ teaspoon cinnamon
- 1½ pound boneless skinless chicken breasts

FOR THE CILANTRO LIME CAULIFLOWER RICE:

- 4 cups cauliflower rice (see note)
- Avocado oil cooking spray
- Sea salt and pepper to taste
- 1 teaspoon lime zest (from 1 lime)
- Juice from 1 lime
- ⅓ cup chopped cilantro

FOR THE MANGO SALSA:

- 1 ripe avocado, diced
- 1 cup mango, cut into ½-inch cubes
- ½ cup halved grape tomatoes
- ¼ cup finely diced red onion
- ¼ cup finely chopped red bell pepper
- ¼ cup chopped cilantro
- 1 tablespoon finely chopped jalapeno (optional)
- Juice from 1 lime
- Sea salt and black pepper to taste

continued

directions

1. Preheat the oven to 400° F. Spray a large oven-safe skillet or cast-iron skillet with cooking spray.

2. To make the jerk seasoning: In a small bowl, combine the garlic powder, onion powder, cayenne pepper, sea salt, black pepper, coconut sugar, dried thyme, paprika, cumin, and cinnamon. Stir to blend. Pat the chicken dry with a paper towel. Evenly rub the jerk seasoning over both sides of the chicken breasts until coated.

3. To make the cauliflower rice: Line a baking sheet with parchment paper. Spread the cauliflower rice evenly on the baking sheet, coat with avocado spray, and season with sea salt and black pepper. Roast for 18–20 minutes. Transfer the cooked cauliflower rice to a large bowl. Add the lime zest, lime juice, and cilantro, and stir to combine. Season with a dash of sea salt if needed.

4. Heat a skillet over medium-high heat. Cook the chicken for 5 minutes on one side, flip, and cook 3 more minutes before transferring the skillet to the oven for 15 to 18 minutes, until the internal temperature of the chicken reaches 165° F. Set aside until ready to plate.

5. To make the mango salsa: In a medium mixing bowl, combine the avocado, mango, grape tomatoes, red onion, red bell pepper, cilantro, jalapeno, lime juice, sea salt, and pepper. Stir until all of the ingredients are blended. Set aside until ready to use.

6. To serve: Divide the cilantro lime cauliflower rice between four plates. Slice the jerk chicken into strips, and distribute it evenly between the plates, placing it on top or beside the cauliflower rice. Spoon the mango salsa on top of the chicken. Garnish with extra cilantro if desired.

notes

» *One 16-ounce bag of pre-riced cauliflower yields 4 cups; otherwise, you can use one head of cauliflower cut into florets. Chop the florets in a food processor until the consistency of rice.*

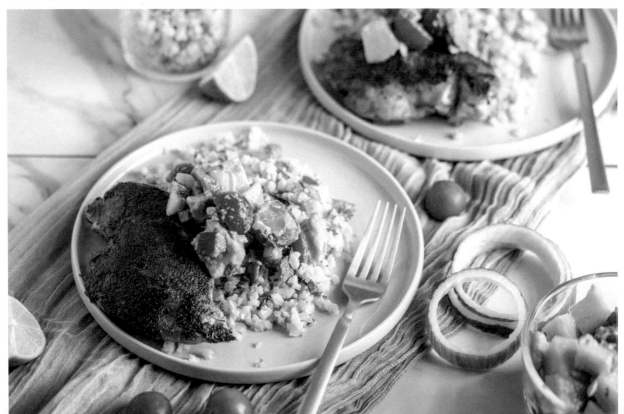

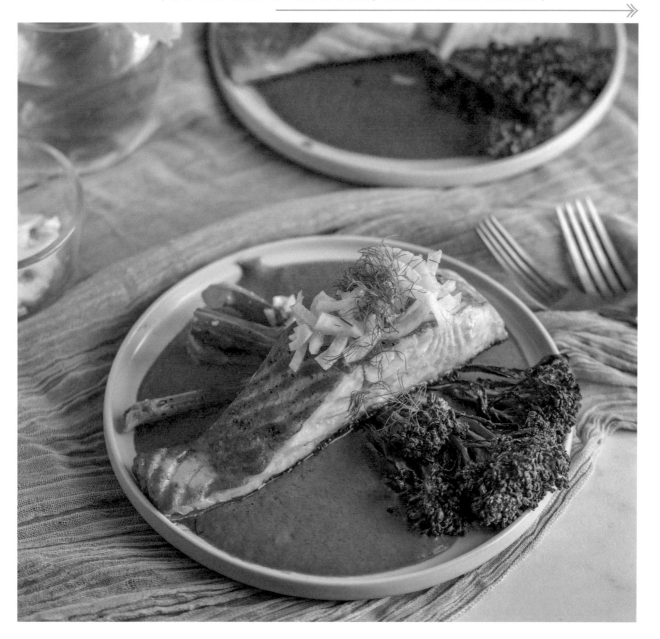

salmon romesco
WITH A CITRUS FENNEL SLAW

Makes 2 servings

My husband and I once dined at a local bar and grill where I ordered the Salmon Romesco. I had never heard of it before, but being someone who gravitates toward seafood, it seemed right up my alley. When it was served, I couldn't help thinking how colorful it was, and I knew I needed to recreate it for this book.

continued

ingredients

FOR THE CITRUS FENNEL SLAW:

- ½ fennel bulb, thinly sliced
- 1 teaspoon thinly sliced (⅛-inch-thick) scallions
- ¼ teaspoon chopped fresh dill
- 1 teaspoon orange zest
- 2 tablespoons fresh orange juice (about ½ orange)
- 1 teaspoon olive oil
- Pinch of coconut sugar (optional)
- Sea salt and black pepper to taste

FOR THE ROMESCO SAUCE:

- 1 red bell pepper, quartered and seeds removed
- Cooking spray
- Dash of sea salt
- ½ cup vegetable or chicken stock
- ½ cup olive oil
- 2 tablespoons tomato paste
- 2 garlic cloves, minced
- ½ teaspoon paprika
- ½ teaspoon sea salt

FOR THE SALMON AND BROCCOLINI:

- 2 (6-ounce) salmon fillets
- 1 small bunch broccolini
- 4 tablespoons avocado oil or coconut oil for cooking, divided (or cooking spray)
- Sea salt and black pepper

directions

1. Preheat the oven to 400° F. Line a baking sheet with parchment paper.

2. Make the citrus fennel slaw: In a medium mixing bowl, combine the sliced fennel, scallions, dill, orange juice, orange zest, olive oil, coconut sugar (if using), sea salt, and pepper. Stir until all of the ingredients are coated in the orange juice. Allow the slaw to marinate in the refrigerator for at least 1 hour.

3. Make the Romesco sauce: Place the red pepper face down on one of the baking sheets and lightly coat with avocado or olive oil and a dash of sea salt. Cook for 30 to 35 minutes, until the red peppers have softened and the edges have started to brown.

4. In a high-speed blender or food processor, combine the roasted bell pepper, stock, olive oil, tomato paste, garlic, paprika, and sea salt. Blend until smooth and creamy. Set aside until ready to plate.

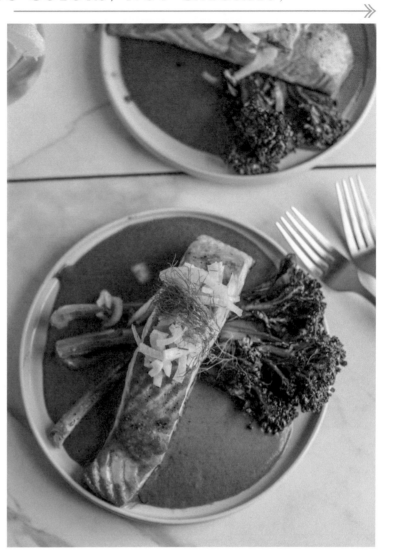

5. Place the broccolini on a baking sheet lined with parchment paper (use the same one you used for roasting the red peppers), coat with oil, and season with sea salt and black pepper. Roast for 20 minutes.

6. Make the salmon: Heat oil in a medium skillet over medium-high heat. Season both sides of the salmon with sea salt and black pepper. Start with the salmon skin side up, and cook 3 to 5 minutes, until slightly golden brown. Flip the salmon and finish off in the oven, cooking 15 to 18 minutes, until the internal temperature reaches 145° F. You can finish in the oven while the broccolini is cooking.

7. To serve, evenly spoon the Romesco sauce onto a shallow bowl or plate. Layer in the broccolini and salmon, and top with the citrus fennel slaw.

note

» *Save the other half of the fennel to roast, or enjoy it raw in a salad or colorful Buddha bowl.*

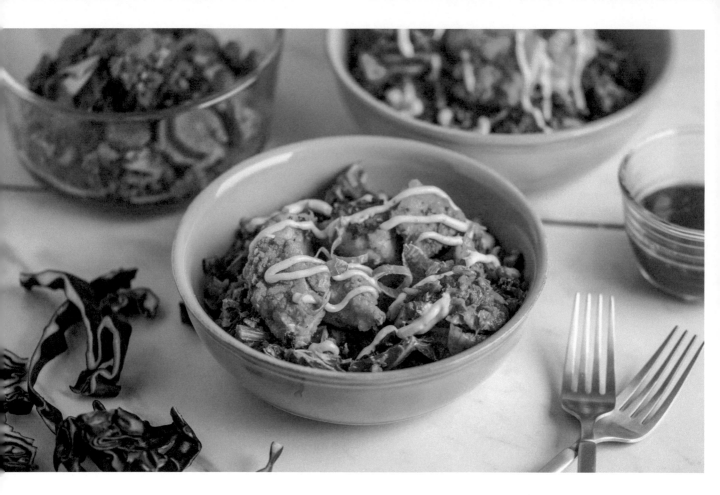

teriyaki chicken kimchi bowls
WITH SPICY MAYO

Makes 4 servings

The inspiration for this recipe came from "Diners, Drive-Ins, and Dives" (fun fact: I am a huge "Triple D" fan!). The segment featured Korean fried chicken kimchi buns with a spicy mayo, and the dish looked delicious. I put a healthier spin on the dish by upgrading some ingredients and using mostly plants. This meal will be a treat for your tastebuds while also making you feel good physically. Additionally, kimchi is not only colorful but is also a gut-friendly fermented food.

ingredients

FOR THE CHICKEN:

- ⅓ cup cassava flour (or gluten-free flour of choice)
- 1 teaspoon sea salt
- 1¼–1½ pounds boneless skinless chicken breasts, cut into 2-inch pieces
- 1 egg, beaten
- ½ cup avocado oil or other cooking oil

FOR THE SRIRACHA AIOLI:

- ⅓ cup avocado mayo (like Primal Kitchen brand)
- 1 teaspoon Sriracha (or hot sauce)

FOR THE TERIYAKI SAUCE:

- ½ cup coconut aminos or tamari
- ¼ cup rice vinegar
- 2 tablespoons maple syrup or coconut nectar
- 1 tablespoon sesame oil
- 3 garlic cloves, minced
- 2 teaspoons freshly grated ginger

FOR THE VEGGIES:

- Cooking spray or oil
- 4 cups cauliflower rice (see note)
- 2 large or medium carrots, peeled and thinly sliced into coins
- 5–6 cups chopped curly kale
- 3 cups shredded or chopped purple cabbage
- 2 scallions (green part only), thinly sliced (plus more for garnish if desired)
- ½–¾ cup kimchi, roughly chopped (depending on desired level of spiciness)

directions

1. Preheat the oven to 400° F. Line a baking sheet with parchment paper.

2. Evenly spread the cauliflower rice and carrot on the baking sheet, and lightly coat with oil or cooking spray. Bake for 20 minutes.

3. Meanwhile, make the chicken: In a large bowl, combine the cassava flour and sea salt. Stir to combine. Place the pieces of chicken in a separate bowl, and pour the beaten egg on top. Allow any excess egg to drip off, and transfer the chicken to the large bowl with the flour mixture. Stir until the chicken is fully coated in the flour mixture.

2. Heat the avocado oil in a large, deep skillet over medium-high heat. Evenly space the chicken in the bottom of the skillet and cook 5 to 6 minutes, until slightly golden brown. Flip each piece of chicken and cook 3 to 4 more minutes, until the internal temperature of the chicken has reached 165° F. Transfer the chicken to a plate or cutting board until ready to serve.

3. Make the teriyaki sauce: In a small bowl, whisk together the coconut aminos or tamari, rice vinegar, maple syrup or coconut nectar, sesame oil, garlic, and ginger.

4. Make the veggies: In a large pot or Dutch oven over medium-high heat, combine the kale, roasted cauliflower rice and carrots, purple cabbage, and scallions. Add the teriyaki sauce and cook about 5 to 6 minutes, until the vegetables have softened and flavors have melded.

5. Make the spicy mayo: In a small bowl, whisk together the mayo and Sriracha.

6. To serve, divide the veggies equally between bowls, then evenly distribute the chicken, and top with kimchi. Spoon or drizzle the spicy mayo on top.

continued

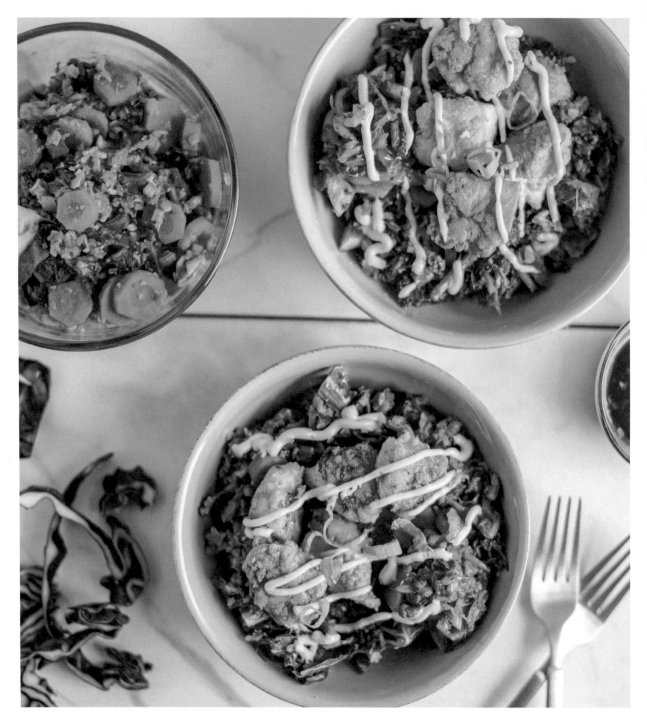

notes

» One 16-ounce bag of pre-riced cauliflower yields 4 cups; otherwise, you can use one head of cauliflower cut into florets. Chop the florets in a food processor until the consistency of rice.

» The first time I made this recipe, I got a pre-made teriyaki stir fry kit at the grocery store and used it for the veggie portion of this recipe. Feel free to do the same if you can find it, keeping in mind that the serving size may be different.

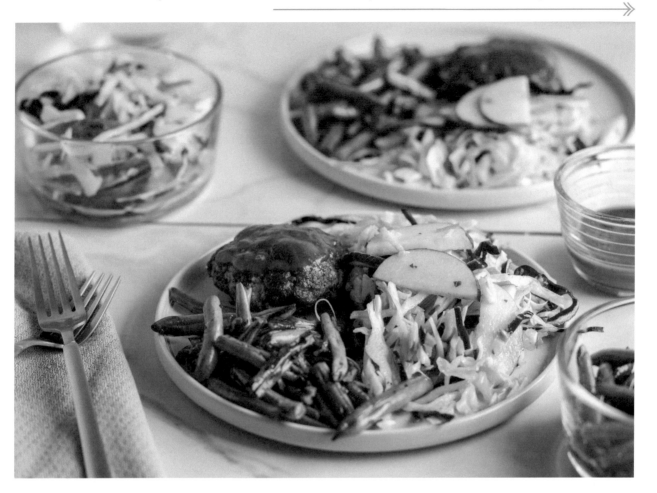

barbecue pork patties

WITH CABBAGE-APPLE SLAW AND GREEN BEANS

Makes 4 servings

This recipe screams the colorful ingredients of summer, but it can really be enjoyed during any season. Barbecue can be a traditionally colorless dish, but not with this recipe. I love eating this meal al fresco in warmer months, or cozied up inside when it is cold.

ingredients

- 1 medium apple, cored and halved (such as Gala or Fuji)
- 1 pound ground pork (or ground beef)
- Sea salt and black pepper
- ½ cup barbecue sauce (like Primal Kitchen brand)

continued »

- ¼ cup olive oil
- Juice from 1 lemon
- 1 tablespoon chopped fresh parsley
- ½ teaspoon ground cumin
- 4–5 cups coleslaw mix (or shredded green and purple cabbage)
- 12 ounces green beans, stems removed and halved widthwise (equals about 5 cups)
- 1 ounce pecans, roughly chopped (equals about ¼ cup)

directions

1. Preheat the oven to 450° F. Line a baking sheet with parchment paper.

2. Grate half of the apple on the large holes of a box grater into a large bowl. Using a paper towel or dish towel, squeeze to remove some of the water (but not all of it). Place it back into the bowl. Lay the remaining half of the apple flat and cut it lengthwise into slices, about ¼ inch thick.

3. Make the pork patties: Add the ground pork to the bowl with the grated apple. Season with sea salt and black pepper. Stir everything together until the ingredients are blended. Use your hands to form patties of equal size, about 3 inches in diameter. Place them on the baking sheet, and evenly spoon the barbecue sauce on top of each one. Bake 15 to 20 minutes, until the patties are fully cooked and reach the internal temperature of 145° F.

4. Make the slaw: In a small bowl, whisk together the olive oil, lemon juice, fresh parsley, ground cumin, and a dash of sea salt and black pepper. Place the coleslaw mix (or shredded cabbage) into a large bowl with the thinly sliced apple. Pour the dressing on top. Set aside to marinate until ready to plate.

5. Sauté the green beans: Heat 1½ to 2 tablespoons of cooking oil in a large skillet over medium-high heat. Season with sea salt and black pepper. Cook 5 to 6 minutes, until the green beans begin to soften, stirring occasionally. Add the pecans, and cook 3 to 4 more minutes, stirring occasionally, until the green beans are tender and pecans are toasted.

6. To serve, place a barbecue pork patty on each plate. Serve with the cabbage-apple slaw and green beans with pecans on the side.

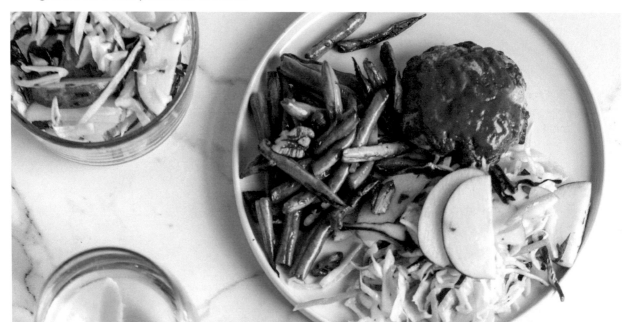

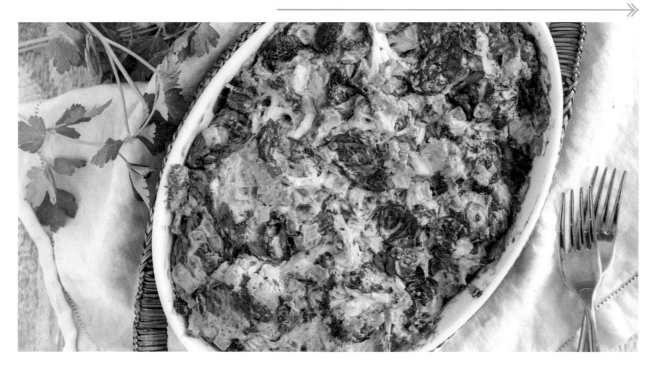

cauliflower, mushroom, & spinach
GRATIN

Serves 6 (as a side), Recipe by Kate Stephenson

Traditionally, a gratin is a dish that is topped with cheese or breadcrumbs and baked until golden brown and crispy. Kate Stephenson was the one who wrote this recipe, and her creative talents are all about using plant-based ingredients that are also good for your gut. Therefore, this colorful gratin uses the power of plants to yield a gluten-free and dairy-free side that is still bubbling with flavor.

ingredients

- 1 head cauliflower, chopped into small florets
- 5 tablespoons olive oil
- Salt and pepper to taste
- 16 ounces cremini or white button mushrooms
- ¾ cup raw cashews, soaked for at least 4–6 hours or overnight, and drained (see note)
- 1 cup vegetable broth or water
- 1 tablespoon coconut aminos (or soy sauce or tamari)
- 1 white or yellow onion, diced
- 2 cloves garlic, minced
- 2 teaspoons chopped fresh thyme leaves
- ¼ cup chopped fresh parsley

continued

- 1 tablespoon chopped fresh oregano
- 5 ounces spinach
- Juice of ½ lemon

directions

1. Preheat the oven to 400° F. Line two baking sheets with parchment paper.

2. Place cauliflower florets in a large mixing bowl. Toss with 2 tablespoons of olive oil, and sea salt and pepper to taste. Spread the florets evenly on the baking sheet and bake for 25 minutes.

3. Meanwhile, prepare the mushrooms: Clean the mushrooms with a wet paper towel. De-stem the mushrooms using your hands but reserve the stems. Quarter the mushrooms and transfer to a mixing bowl (you can use the same bowl as the cauliflower). Roughly chop the stems and transfer them to the bowl as well. Toss with 2 tablespoons olive oil, and salt and pepper to taste.

4. Spread the mushrooms onto the second baking sheet and bake for 10 minutes until the mushrooms have some color and have released their moisture. You can time this step with the final 10 minutes of baking the cauliflower florets.

5. Once done cooking, transfer the cauliflower and mushrooms back to the mixing bowl. I suggest using a slotted spoon to transfer the mushrooms so the liquid stays in the pan and does not transfer to the bowl. Toss together and set aside.

6. Turn down the oven to 375° F. Prepare a 2-quart casserole dish. Drizzle a bit of olive oil in the bottom of the dish and swirl it around so it covers most of the bottom, or coat with cooking spray.

7. Place the soaked cashews in a high-speed blender. Add vegetable broth and coconut aminos, and blend on high until the cashews are completely smooth.

8. Heat 1 tablespoon olive oil in a large sauté pan over medium-low heat. Transfer the diced onion to the pan along with a pinch of salt, and sauté for 5 to 7 minutes, until softened. Add in minced garlic and sauté for another minute until fragrant.

9. Pour the cashew mixture into the pan and combine with onions and garlic. Add in chopped herbs, and stir to combine. Bring the mixture to a low simmer and continue to stir until it starts to thicken. Taste, and add more salt and pepper if needed.

10. With the temperature low, add in the spinach; add it in batches if necessary. Stir until it is almost wilted, about 3 to 5 minutes.

11. Squeeze in the lemon juice, and stir into the mixture.

12. Pour the cauliflower and mushroom mixture into the pan, and turn off the heat. Stir everything to combine. Taste, and add more salt and pepper if necessary. Transfer the mixture to the casserole dish.

13. Bake for 20 to 25 minutes, until lightly browned and bubbling.

notes

» *If short on time, you can prepare the soaked cashews 30 minutes to an hour ahead of cooking by using boiling water. Place cashews in a medium mixing bowl and cover with boiling water. Allow them to soak for 30 minutes to 1 hour. Drain.*

» *For extra greens, add a layer of spinach to the bottom of the casserole dish before adding the cauliflower mushroom mixture in Step 12.*

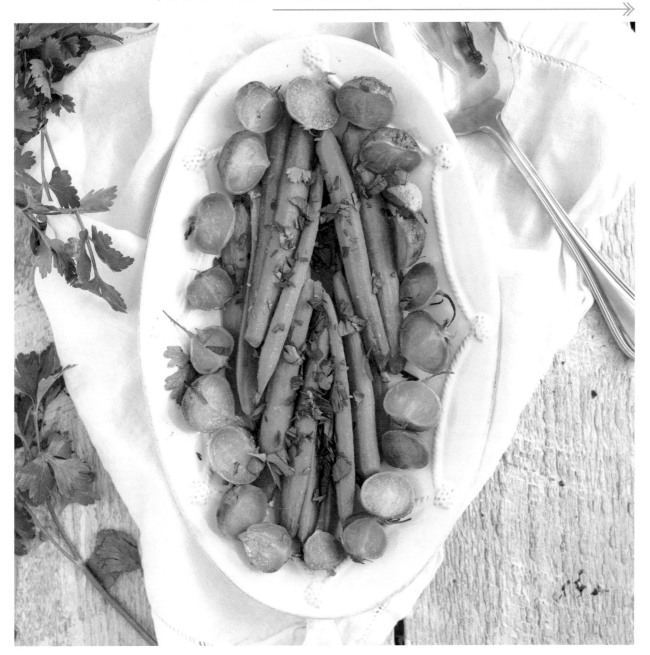

orange roasted
CARROTS AND RADISHES

Serves 4 (as a side), Recipe by Kate Stephenson

Radishes are so beautiful in color yet can have a bitter taste when eaten raw (hint: bitter vegetables are packed with nutrition!). However, when you roast them in a flavorful dressing, like the one found below, they are delicious, especially when paired with a sweet vegetable like carrots.

continued

ingredients

- 1 bunch of carrots (about 8–10 medium carrots)
- 1 bunch of radishes (about 4–5 radishes)
- ¼ teaspoon ground cumin
- 3 teaspoons honey
- Zest from ½ orange
- Juice from ½ orange
- 1 tablespoon avocado oil
- ½ teaspoon salt
- ¼ teaspoon black pepper
- 1 small handful of parsley or cilantro, roughly chopped

directions

1. Preheat the oven to 400° F. Line a baking sheet with parchment paper.

2. Prep the carrots and radishes: Peel the carrots and either leave them whole or slice them lengthwise down the center. The carrots should be around the same size for even cooking, so you may need to leave the small carrots whole and slice the larger carrots.

3. Remove the tops from the radishes and wash them. Quarter or halve the radishes depending on their size. Transfer all veggies to a large mixing bowl.

4. In a small bowl, combine the cumin, honey, orange zest, orange juice, oil, salt, and pepper.

5. Drizzle the dressing over the carrots and radishes, and use your hands to toss everything together.

6. Spread the carrots and radishes in an even layer onto the baking sheet.

7. Bake for 18 to 20 minutes, until the carrots and radishes have some color. They should be fork tender but not mushy.

8. Transfer the carrots and radishes to a serving platter. Sprinkle with herbs.

note

» *Zest your orange before juicing.*

purple sweet potato
AND CARROT SOUP

Makes 4 servings

This purple sweet potato and carrot soup is one of my earliest Counting Colors recipes. When I started to eat more whole, real foods, my mom had sent me a newspaper clipping (yes, a newspaper clipping) for a sweet potato carrot ginger soup. After discovering the purple varieties in the produce section, I made the substitution, and this vibrant version was born. Sitting down with a bowl of this colorful soup is playful for the eyes and comforting for the soul.

ingredients

- 4 cups vegetable stock or chicken stock
- 5 purple carrots, peeled and chopped (equals about 2 cups)
- 2 purple sweet potatoes, peeled and diced (equals about 4–5 cups)
- 2 teaspoons grated ginger
- ½ teaspoon ground cinnamon
- ¼ teaspoon sea salt, plus more to taste
- Pinch of cayenne pepper to taste (optional)
- Black pepper to taste

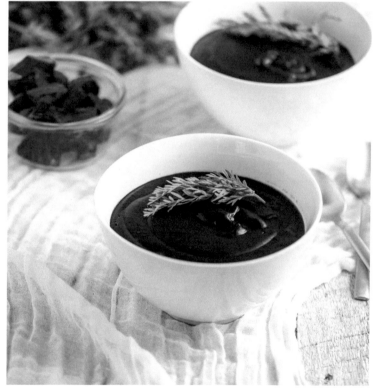

directions

1. In a large pot or Dutch oven, combine the stock, chopped carrots, and diced sweet potatoes. Cover the pot with the lid and bring to a boil. Reduce the heat to a low simmer, and cook for 10 minutes.

2. Add the ginger, cinnamon, sea salt, cayenne, and black pepper. Place the lid back on the pot, and cook 15 more minutes, until flavors have melded and vegetables are fork tender.

3. Remove the pot from heat. Using an immersion blender, process until a smooth, creamy consistency. You can also transfer the soup to a high-speed blender and process in batches. Serve warm.

note

» *You can use regular carrots and sweet potato for this recipe, just know that the color will be orange and not purple. This change would still yield a colorful and nutritious option!*

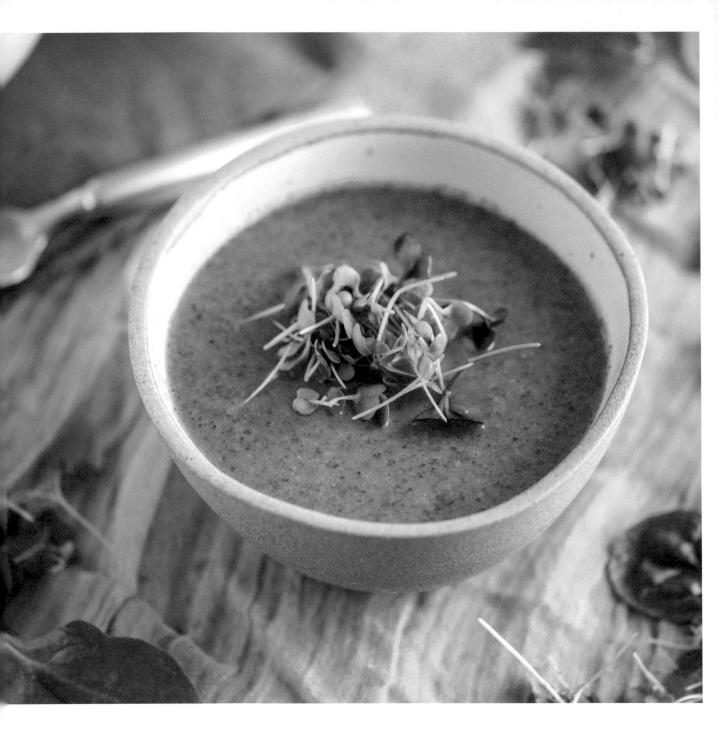

green reset soup

Makes 3 to 4 servings (about 5 cups total)

This veggie-heavy and nutrient-dense soup is perfect for when you want to give your digestive system a break. The fiber found in the vegetables also helps keep you full, while the ginger and turmeric support your natural detoxification pathways. The green color of this soup lets you know how nourishing it truly is.

ingredients

- 1 tablespoon ghee or coconut oil for cooking
- 1 yellow onion, diced (equals about 1 cup)
- Sea salt and black pepper to taste
- 1 clove garlic, minced
- 1 teaspoon grated ginger
- 1 medium zucchini, chopped into 1-inch chunks (equals about 2 cups)
- 1 cup cauliflower florets
- 1 cup broccoli florets
- 3 cups vegetable stock
- 3 cups organic spinach
- 1 cup loosely packed and chopped parsley
- 1 teaspoon turmeric
- Microgreens for garnish (optional)

directions

1. Heat ghee or coconut oil in a large soup pot or Dutch oven over medium heat. Add diced yellow onion. Season with sea salt and cook until fragrant and slightly browned, about 4 minutes, stirring occasionally. Add in garlic and ginger, and sauté for an additional 1 to 2 minutes, stirring frequently to prevent burning.

2. Add zucchini, cauliflower, and broccoli, and season with sea salt and black pepper. Stir everything together and cook 1 to 2 minutes.

3. Add the vegetable stock and increase the heat to high. Cover the soup pot with a lid and bring it to boil.

4. Give the soup a good stir, reduce the heat to a low simmer, and cook 20 more minutes uncovered, until vegetables are fork tender. Add the spinach, parsley, turmeric, and sea salt and black pepper to taste, stirring until the greens start to wilt and are incorporated, about 1 minute.

5. Turn off the heat. Blend the soup with an immersion hand blender or transfer the soup in batches to a high-speed blender and process until creamy and smooth. Taste and adjust seasoning as necessary. Divide the soup evenly between bowls, and top with microgreens if desired. Serve warm.

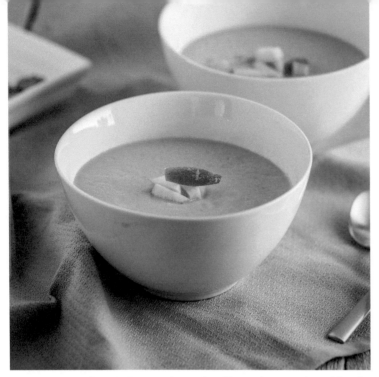

cauliflower & apple soup

Makes about 6 cups or 4 servings

This recipe dates back to my early blogging days. During this time, I was trying to reduce the processed foods in my diet and consume more whole fruits and vegetables instead. It was one of the first healthy recipes I tried, tested, and posted. The combination of cauliflower and apple pleasantly surprised me, and I was amazed at how creamy and delicious it was; not to mention, it is easy to make. The color may be white (arguably not a color), but hear me out: In my opinion, when it comes to nutrition and whole foods found in nature, white is a color. Cauliflower is high in vitamins C, K, and B6; it is also a good source of fiber and folate. It is a cruciferous vegetable, which is a family of plants known to help lower inflammation.

ingredients

- 1 small to medium head of cauliflower, chopped into small florets (equals about 6 cups)
- 3 medium apples, cored and diced (like Gala or Fuji, plus more for topping if desired)
- 1 cup water (plus more for steaming the cauliflower)
- 1 tablespoon olive oil
- 1 tablespoon apple cider vinegar
- ¼ teaspoon sea salt
- Black pepper to taste

directions

1. Steam the cauliflower: Place the cauliflower florets in a large skillet over high heat. Place enough water in the skillet to slightly cover the florets (about halfway covered, not covered completely). Cover the skillet with a lid and bring the water to a boil. Reduce the heat to a simmer and cook until the cauliflower is fork tender, about 7 to 10 minutes. Drain the cauliflower and place it in a high-speed blender.

2. Add the apple, water, olive oil, apple cider vinegar, sea salt, and black pepper to the blender. Process until creamy and warm, about 2 minutes. If you don't have a high-speed blender (such as a Vitamix), you can process the soup ingredients in a food processor (in batches if needed), and enjoy as is, or place the processed ingredients in a soup pot to warm through.

3. Divide the soup into bowls, and top with extra diced apple if desired.

this color
CAN'T BE BEET SOUP

Makes 4 servings

Beets can be an acquired taste, but they sure are beautiful. The color of this soup is hard to beet (see what I did there?). With an earthy yet sweet and creamy taste and texture, you know you are eating something beneficial for your health. This soup will not only satiate you but will also be a feast for your eyes.

ingredients

- 2 tablespoons avocado or olive oil
- 2 white or yellow onions, peeled and diced
- 2 garlic cloves, minced
- 1 tablespoon freshly grated ginger
- 3 large beets, stems removed, peeled, and diced (use 4 if they are smaller)
- 1 medium parsnip or carrot, peeled and diced (yields about 1 cup)
- 4 cups vegetable stock
- ¼ teaspoon sea salt and black pepper, or more to taste
- Coconut cream or coconut yogurt and parsley for garnish if desired

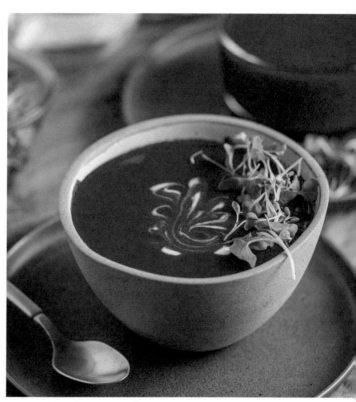

directions

1. Heat oil in a large soup pot or Dutch oven over medium-high heat. Add the diced onion and cook 4 to 5 minutes stirring occasionally, until the onion starts to soften and turn golden brown.

2. Add the minced garlic and grated ginger to the pot. Cook for an additional 2 to 3 minutes, stirring frequently.

3. Add the diced beets, diced parsnip or carrot, and stir to combine the vegetables with the rest of the ingredients. Season with some sea salt and black pepper, and stir. Add the vegetable stock. Turn the heat to high and bring to a boil. Reduce the heat to low, cover the pot, and simmer for 30 minutes, or until the beets and parsnip or carrot are fork tender.

4. Use an immersion blender to process the soup until creamy. If you don't have an immersion blender, you can transfer the soup to a high-speed blender or food processor (in batches if needed) and process until smooth.

5. Divide the soup between bowls. Garnish with coconut cream or yogurt and parsley if desired. Serve warm.

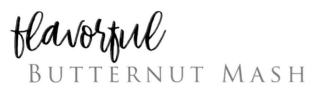

flavorful
BUTTERNUT MASH

Makes 4 servings

This mashed butternut squash dates back to my early recipe-creating days. I would always get so inspired when I discovered new ingredients to play around with and enjoy. White miso and nutritional yeast are prime examples, and when used together they yield the most delicious flavor (hence the name). You can of course make this recipe without them for a more basic butternut mash, but I highly encourage you incorporate them for more flavor.

ingredients

- 3–4 cups butternut squash, diced into 1-inch cubes (see note)
- 2 tablespoons nutritional yeast
- 1 tablespoon white miso (chickpea or brown rice miso, but soy miso will also work)
- 2 teaspoons Dijon or brown mustard
- ½ teaspoon garlic powder
- ½ teaspoon onion powder
- ½ teaspoon sea salt (plus more to taste)

directions

1. Preheat the oven to 400° F. Line a baking sheet with parchment paper. Spread the diced butternut squash evenly on the baking sheet, and roast 25 to 30 minutes, until fork tender.

2. Transfer the squash to a large mixing bowl. Add the nutritional yeast, miso, mustard, garlic powder, onion powder, and sea salt. Use an immersion blender or a potato masher until all of the ingredients are blended together and the consistency is slightly creamy. You can also add all ingredients to a food processor and blend. There might still be some butternut squash chunks, but that is OK.

3. Stir everything in the bowl with a spatula, and blend again if needed; or scrape down the bowl of the food processor and pulse as needed. Serve warm.

note

» *The quantity of 3–4 cups butternut squash equals about one medium butternut squash or one store-bought box of pre-diced butternut squash cubes.*

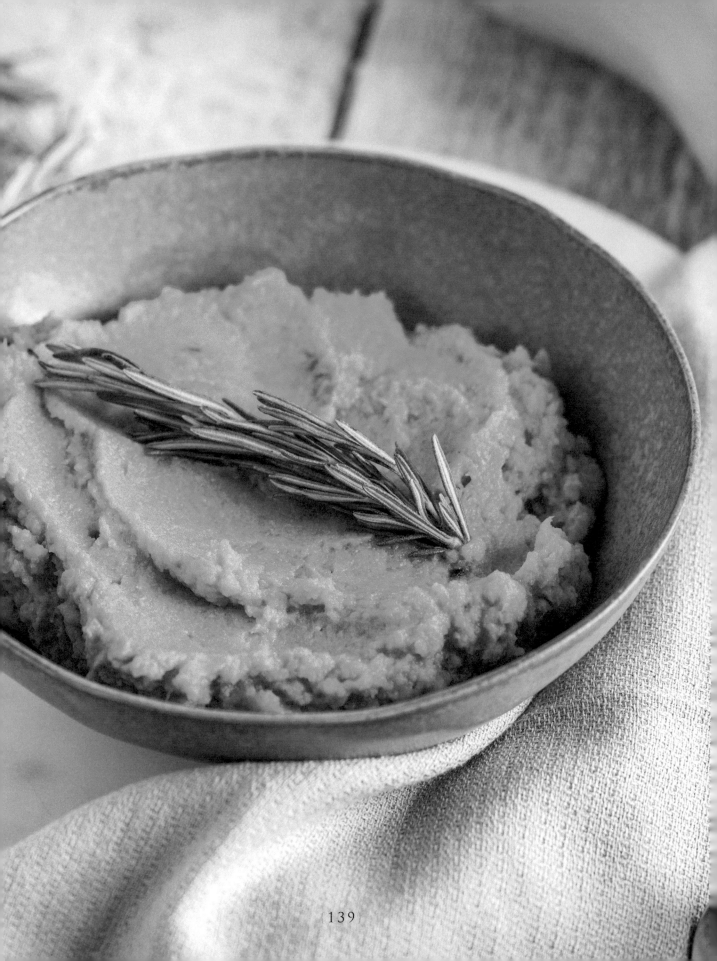

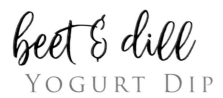

beet & dill
YOGURT DIP

Makes 8 ounces
Recipe by Kate Stephenson

You will wow your guests, friends, or family when you present them with this beet and dill yogurt dip. The dish is bold and beautiful in color, while also being delicious and packed with nutrition. A slight sweetness is balanced nicely by dill and yogurt flavors. Serve with raw vegetables or grain-free crackers on the side.

ingredients

- 2 small or 1 medium beet (equals about 1 cup)
- ½ cup plain unsweetened coconut yogurt (or any plain unsweetened yogurt)
- ½ teaspoon minced garlic
- 2 teaspoons honey
- 2 tablespoons olive oil
- 2 teaspoons red wine vinegar
- 1 teaspoon salt
- 2 tablespoons chopped fresh dill
- ⅓ cup whole raw walnuts (optional)

directions

1. Peel the beet and transfer to a small pot. Cover with water and bring to a boil. Cook until the beet is very fork tender (about 30 to 40 minutes). Transfer to a colander and rinse with water. When the beet is cool enough to handle, roughly chop the beet. There should be about 1 cup of chopped beets total. Allow the beets to cool.

2. Combine the cooked, chopped beets, yogurt, garlic, honey, olive oil, red wine vinegar, and salt in a high-speed blender or food processor. Mix on high for 1 minute, until the mixture is completely smooth.

3. Transfer the dip to a bowl or container, and fold in the chopped dill.

4. If using walnuts, preheat oven to 350° F. Spread the walnuts onto a baking sheet and toast for 6 to 7 minutes until browned. Let the walnuts slightly cool, about 10 minutes.

5. Transfer the walnuts to a cutting board and roughly chop. Sprinkle the walnuts over the beet dip. Serve.

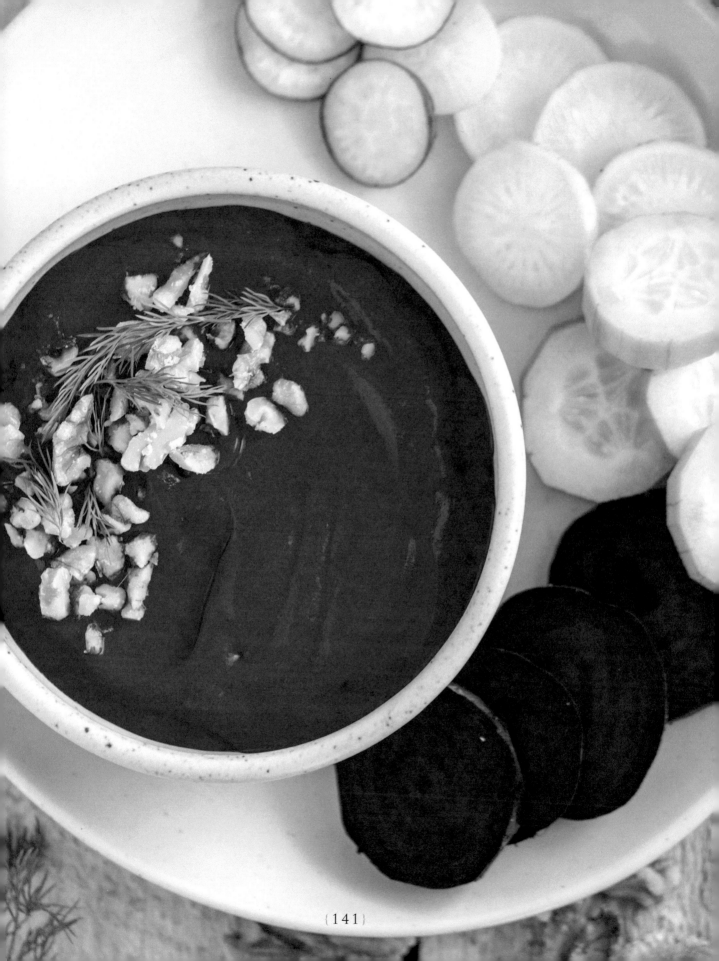

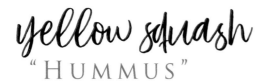

yellow squash
"HUMMUS"

Makes 2 cups

Instead of chickpeas, this dip uses yellow squash as its base. The consistency is similar to the traditional spread, and the vegetable substitution offers vibrant color, as well as vitamin C, potassium, folate, and vitamin B6, to name a few. It is especially great if you are intolerant to legumes or living a lower-carb lifestyle.

ingredients

- 5 cups yellow squash, chopped into 1-inch chunks (equals 3–4 medium squash)
- ¼ cup tahini
- 2 tablespoons olive oil
- Juice from ½ lemon
- 2 cloves garlic, minced
- ½ teaspoon sea salt
- ½ teaspoon cumin (optional)

directions

1. Preheat the oven to 400° F. Line a baking sheet with parchment paper.

2. Spread the squash evenly on the baking sheet and dry-roast until fork tender, about 28 to 30 minutes. Allow the squash to slightly cool, about 10 minutes.

3. Transfer the cooked squash to a food processor or high-speed blender. Add the tahini, olive oil, lemon juice, garlic cloves, sea salt, and cumin (if using). Blend until smooth.

4. Transfer the mixture to a bowl to cool to room temperature. You can enjoy as is, or place the dip in an airtight container in the refrigerator to further chill. The dip is even better the next day!

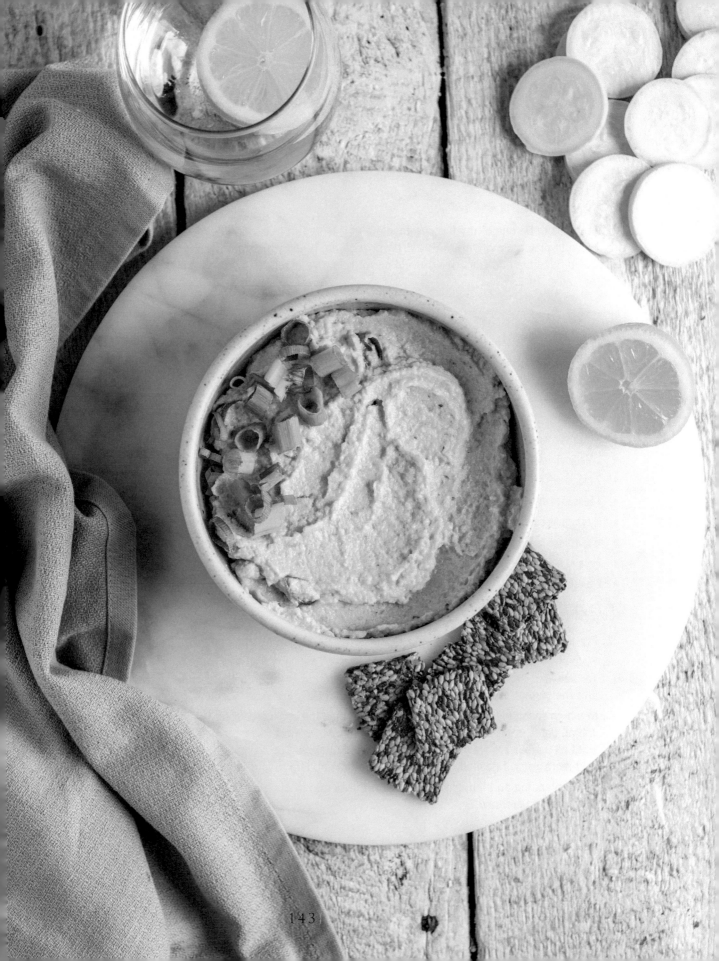

curried carrot
HUMMUS

Makes 24 ounces
Recipe by Kate Stephenson

Hummus has to be one of my favorite foods, and it is so fun to expand beyond the traditional dip. I love to play around with different flavor profiles. When you add other vegetables to the mix, the possibilities are endless. This curried carrot hummus is a great option for choosing your own hummus adventure.

ingredients

- 1 pound carrots, peeled and chopped into 1-inch chunks
- ¾ cup + 1 tablespoon of olive oil, divided
- ½–¾ cup water (see note)
- 1 (13.5-ounce) can of chickpeas, drained and rinsed
- 2 tablespoons tahini
- 2 Medjool dates, pitted
- 2 teaspoons maple syrup
- 1 teaspoon curry powder
- ½ teaspoon cumin
- ½ teaspoon red pepper flakes
- Juice of ½ lemon
- 2 teaspoons sea salt

directions

1. Preheat the oven to 375° F. Line a baking sheet with parchment paper.

2. Spread the carrots evenly onto the baking sheet. Drizzle with 1 tablespoon of olive oil and stir (or use your hands) to coat. Bake for 30 to 35 minutes, or until the carrots are very fork tender. Set the carrots aside to slightly cool, about 15 to 20 minutes.

3. In a high-speed blender or food processor, combine the cooked carrots, ½ cup of water, chickpeas, tahini, dates, maple syrup, curry powder, cumin, red pepper flakes, lemon juice, and sea salt. Blend until all ingredients are starting to incorporate but are not quite smooth. Check the consistency, and add more water if needed, 1 tablespoon at a time and up to four additional tablespoons.

4. While blending on high, slowly drizzle in the ¾ cup of olive oil until everything is blended together and creamy.

note

» *Depending on if you like your hummus chunky or smooth, start with ½ cup of water, and increase up to ¾ cup, 1 tablespoon at a time.*

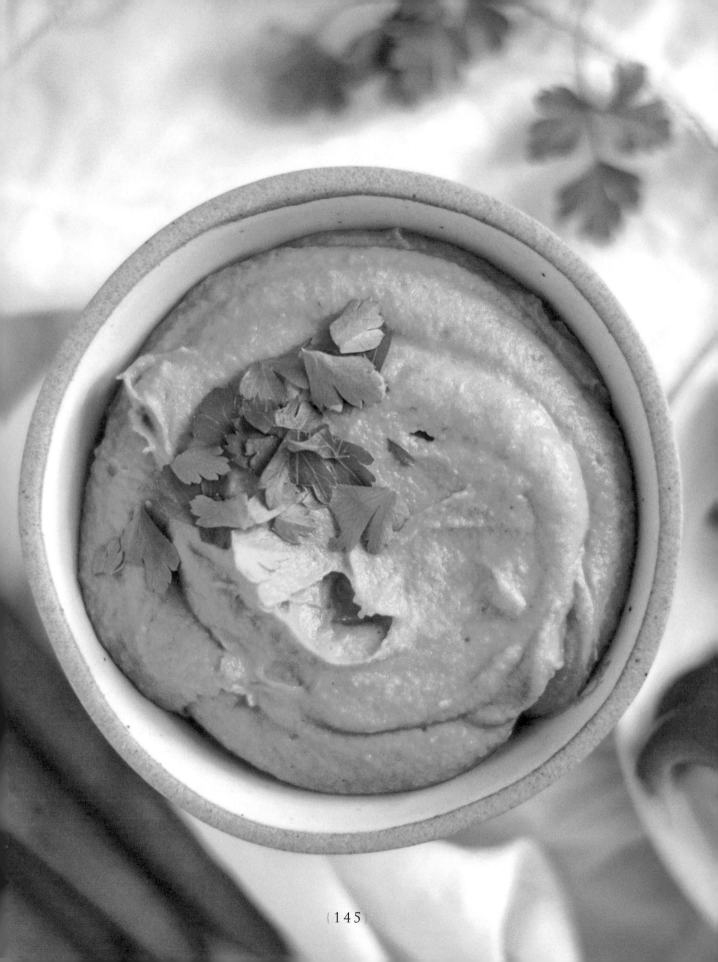

lima bean

DIP

Makes 10 ounces
Recipe by Kate Stephenson

Growing up, lima beans were one of my father's favorite foods. Because of this, my mom felt compelled to serve them often, more often that I would have liked (let's just say they were not my favorite). To encourage me to eat them, he would play a game where whoever fit the most lima beans on their fork, won (anyone else?). Then you had to eat what was on your fork. It did the trick (because clearly, I was tricked). I honestly don't think I ate another lima bean until Kate made this dip. It won me over and changed my opinion about lima beans for good.

ingredients

- 1 cup uncooked lima beans
- 2 tablespoons chopped fresh chives
- Juice of ½ lemon
- ¼ cup parsley leaves
- 2 teaspoons diced shallots (or substitute with minced garlic)
- ½ teaspoon sea salt
- ⅓ cup olive oil

directions

1. Bring a small pot of water to a boil, and cook the lima beans for 8 to 10 minutes. Drain and rinse with cold water. Allow the lima beans to cool for 10 to 15 minutes.

2. In a high-speed blender or food processor, combine the cooked lima beans, chives, lemon juice, parsley, diced shallot, and sea salt. Pulse until all of the ingredients are blended together.

3. With the blender or food processor going, slowly drizzle in the olive oil until the dip is thick and chunky. If you prefer a smoother dip, continue to blend, and add more oil 1 teaspoon at a time until the desired consistency is reached. Taste and adjust seasoning if necessary.

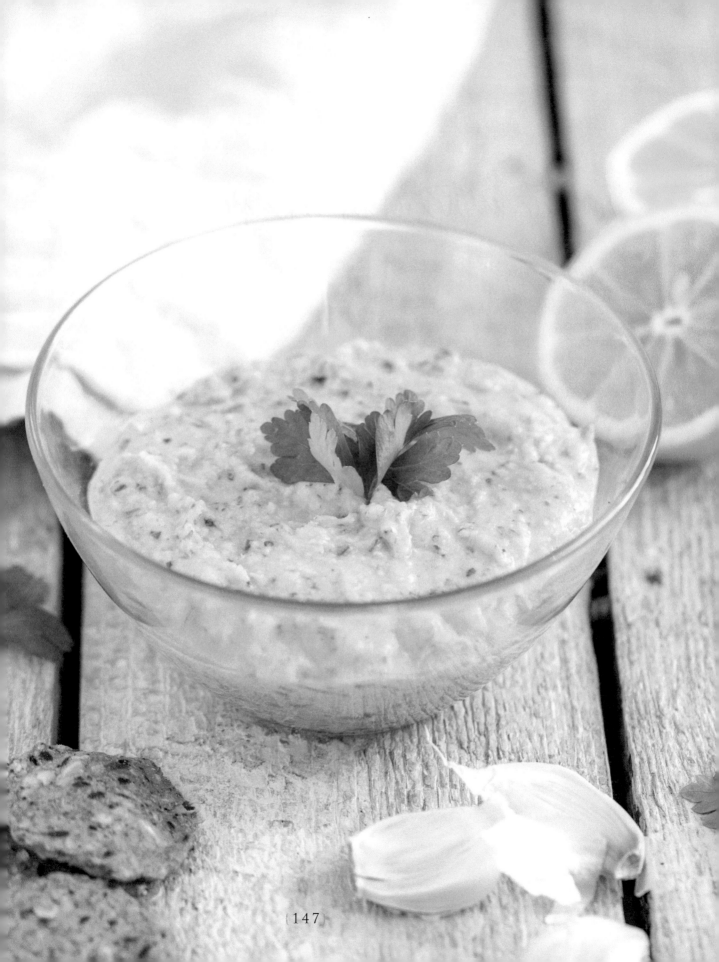

tomato, artichoke, & caper
TAPENADE

Makes 12 ounces
Recipe by Kate Stephenson

There is something about a Mediterranean flavor combination that makes you feel healthy and light on the other side of eating it; this appetizer is no exception. The trifecta of tomatoes, artichokes, and capers in this tapenade will have your tastebuds doing a happy dance. Use as a spread on bruschetta or enjoy as a dip before dinner.

ingredients

- 1 (14-ounce) can artichoke hearts
- 2 tablespoons capers, drained
- 2 cloves garlic
- Zest from ½ lemon
- Juice from ½ lemon
- ⅓ cup chopped parsley
- 1 teaspoon dried oregano
- ½ teaspoon red pepper flakes
- Sea salt and black pepper to taste
- ½ cup chopped cherry tomatoes

directions

1. In a food processor, combine the artichoke hearts, capers, garlic, lemon zest, lemon juice, parsley, dried oregano, red pepper flakes, sea salt, and black pepper to taste. Pulse until the mixture resembles a chunky consistency (it should not be a smooth paste).

2. Transfer the mixture to a mixing bowl and fold in the chopped cherry tomatoes. Taste and adjust the seasoning if necessary.

note

» *Remember to zest your lemon before juicing.*

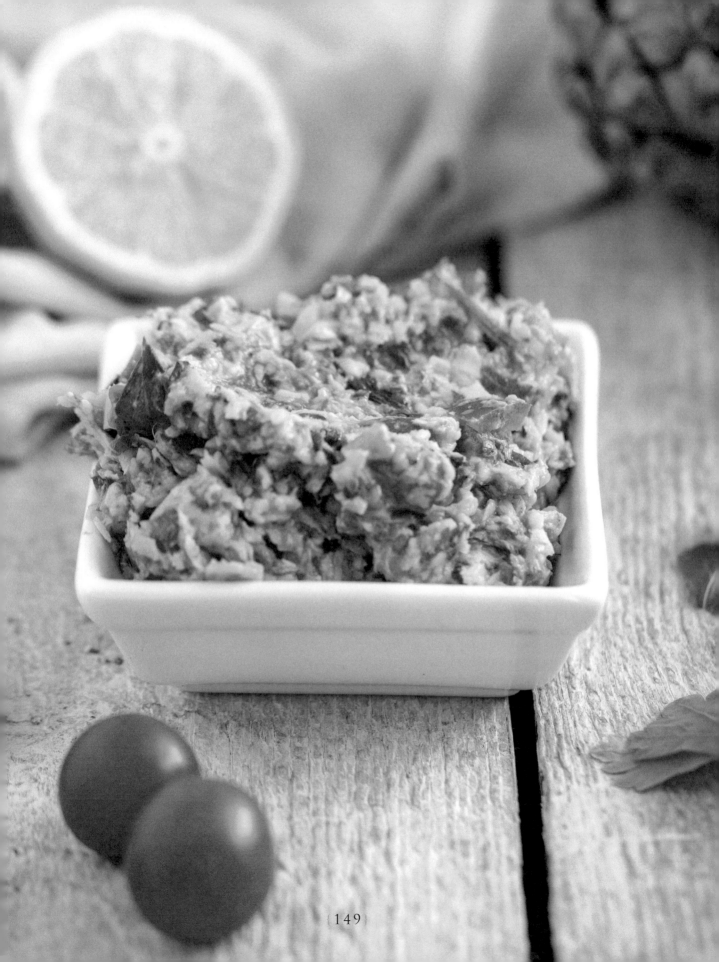

mango jalapeno
SALSA

Makes 2 cups
Recipe by Kate Stephenson

If you like sweet and savory, you will love this salsa. Mango is such an amazing addition to salsa, and it helps to balance out the spice. Plus, it makes it more colorful.

ingredients

- 1 cup diced tomatoes
- ⅔ cup diced mango
- ¼ cup finely chopped red onion
- 2 tablespoons finely chopped jalapeno
- 1 tablespoon finely chopped parsley
- 1 tablespoon finely chopped cilantro
- Zest of ½ lime
- Juice of 1 lime
- ¼ teaspoon sea salt

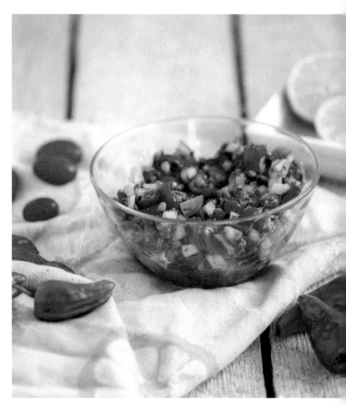

directions

1. Combine all of the ingredients in a medium bowl, and stir to combine. Taste and adjust the seasoning if necessary.

notes

» *Remember to zest your half lime before juicing.*
» *This recipe would also work well with peaches instead of mango.*

sweet potato miso ginger
DIP

Makes 12 ounces, Recipe by Kate Stephenson

This dip was love at first bite. It incorporates my favorite food (sweet potatoes) alongside a few of my favorite flavors. I never would have thought to put them all together, but thankfully, Kate knew what she was doing when she wrote this recipe. This has entered my entertaining rotation when it comes to what to serve or contribute for a gathering or potluck.

ingredients

- 1 medium sweet potato, peeled and cut into 1-inch chunks
- 2 tablespoons olive oil
- 1 tablespoon miso paste (white, brown, or chickpea)
- 1 tablespoon tahini
- 2 teaspoons coconut aminos
- 2 teaspoons rice vinegar
- 2 teaspoons orange zest (from about ½ orange)
- ½ teaspoon freshly grated ginger
- ½ teaspoon red pepper flakes
- 1 teaspoon sea salt
- Cilantro, scallions, and/or sesame seeds for garnish (optional)

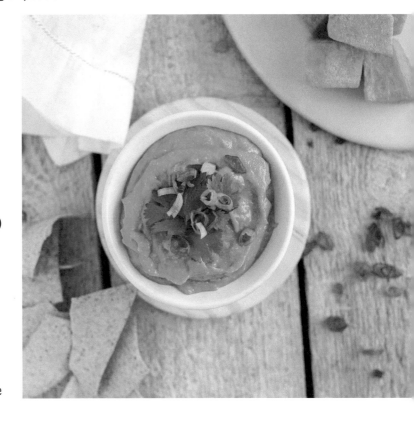

directions

1. Dry-roast the sweet potato: Preheat the oven to 400° F. Line a baking sheet with parchment paper.

2. Spread the sweet potato evenly on the baking sheet and cook for 25 to 30 minutes, until fork tender. Set aside to slightly cool, about 10 to 15 minutes.

3. In a food processor, combine the cooked sweet potato, olive oil, miso paste, tahini, coconut aminos, rice vinegar, orange zest, ginger, red pepper flakes, and sea salt. Blend until very smooth, scraping down the sides of the food processor and pulsing as needed.

4. Transfer the dip to a serving bowl. Garnish with cilantro, scallions, and/or sesame seeds if desired.

note

» *You can use tamari or soy sauce instead of the coconut aminos, but that would no longer make this recipe soy-free or gluten-free (if soy sauce is used).*

strawberry basil
POPSICLES

Makes about 12 medium popsicles

The combination of strawberry and basil tastes like summer, with the majority of the sweetness coming from nature's candy (the fruit!). These popsicles are low-glycemic, nutritious, and refreshing. And with only five ingredients, they are easy to make.

ingredients

- 1 (13.5-ounce) can of full-fat coconut milk
- 3–4 cups whole, fresh strawberries, stems removed (equals about 1 pound)
- ¼ cup maple syrup, honey, or coconut nectar
- 1 teaspoon vanilla extract
- ⅓ cup loosely packed torn basil leaves

directions

1. Add all of the ingredients to a high-speed blender or food processor and blend until smooth, about 30 seconds. Pour the mixture evenly into each popsicle mold, and transfer to the freezer. Allow the popsicles to set, at least 4 to 6 hours or, ideally, overnight.

note

» *You can use frozen strawberries, but given this recipe calls for full-fat coconut milk, I would recommend thawing the strawberries before blending.*

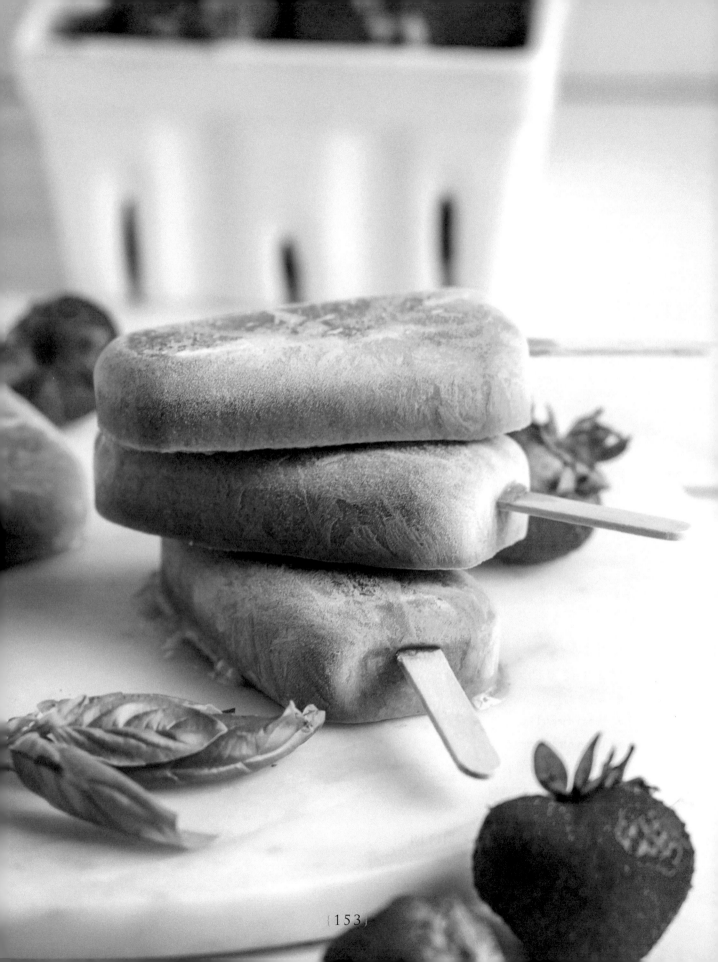

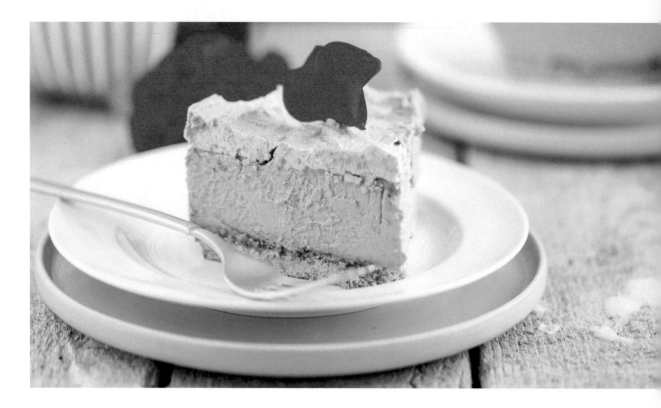

pretty in pink
CHEESECAKE

Makes 10 to 12 servings

This recipe came to be as a result of two reasons: I once found beet root powder at my local natural market and was intrigued. I didn't have an intention for it at the time, but knew I would dream up a recipe eventually. Secondly, as I was finishing this book, colorful desserts were (of course) on my mind. Ta-da! This grain-free and vegan (primarily no-bake) cheesecake was born! I am so happy with how it turned out. It almost has a strawberry ice cream flavor—natural with a hint of sweetness.

ingredients

FOR THE CRUST:

- ½ cup cassava flour
- ½ cup coconut flour
- ¼ cup coconut sugar
- 2 tablespoons arrowroot starch or tapioca flour
- ¼ cup melted coconut oil
- ¼ cup maple syrup

FOR THE CHEESECAKE FILLING:

- ¾ cup full-fat coconut milk
- 2 cups raw cashews, soaked 4–6 hours or overnight (see note)

- 2 ripe medium bananas, mashed (equals about ¾ cup)
- ½ cup coconut cream
- 1 (8-ounce) package vegan cream cheese, softened to room temperature
- ½ cup maple syrup
- 1 tablespoon beet root powder
- 1 teaspoon vanilla extract
- 2 tablespoons melted coconut oil

FOR THE FROSTING (OPTIONAL):

- ½ cup coconut oil, room temperature
- ½ cup palm oil shortening, grass-fed butter, or vegan butter, room temperature
- 2 tablespoon powdered monk fruit (substitute with regular powdered sugar or coconut sugar)
- 1 tablespoon arrowroot starch or tapioca starch
- 1½ teaspoon beet root powder
- 2 tablespoons maple syrup
- 1 teaspoon vanilla extract

directions

1. Preheat the oven to 350° F. Spray an 8-inch round spring-form cake pan with cooking spray.

2. Make the crust: In a large bowl or stand mixer, mix the cassava flour, coconut flour, coconut sugar, and arrowroot starch. Stir to blend. In a separate small bowl, whisk together the melted coconut oil and maple syrup. Pour the wet ingredients into the bowl with the dry ingredients.

3. Start beating on medium speed, increasing the speed and continuing to beat until a crumbly dough is formed. The dough should be the consistency of damp, coarse sand. Gather the dough and press it firmly into the bottom of the cake pan. Bake for 10 to 12 minutes, and then set aside to cool, about 20 to 30 minutes.

4. Meanwhile, make the filling: In a high-speed blender, mix the coconut milk, soaked cashews, mashed banana, coconut cream, vegan cream cheese, maple syrup, beet root powder, and vanilla extract. Blend until creamy, using the tamper as needed to get the blender going and until everything is smooth. Add the melted coconut oil and blend again.

5. Pour the filling mixture into the cake pan with the crust. Transfer the cheesecake to the refrigerator to set, at least 12 hours or, ideally, overnight, for up to 24 hours. Serve and enjoy, or make the frosting.

6. To make the frosting: In a large mixing bowl, combine the coconut oil and palm oil shortening or butter. Beat with a hand mixer until fluffy, about 1 minute.

7. Add the powdered monk fruit, beet root powder, and arrowroot starch, and beat again. Add the maple syrup and vanilla, and beat until everything is combined, using a spatula to scrape down the sides as needed.

8. Using a spatula, mix the frosting. Use the frosting immediately, spreading it evenly on top of the set and chilled cheesecake. Enjoy immediately (if you put it back in the fridge, the frosting will harden, but it is still delicious!).

glazed carrot cake
TRUFFLES

Makes 10 (1½-inch) truffles

I once found some raw carrot cake "muffins" in a juice bar while visiting Chicago. They were so delicious yet made with the simplest ingredients. It was my first foray into the world of healthier sweets. It was then that I learned you could satisfy your sugar cravings with desserts made with upgraded ingredients, and sometimes, no baking is needed! I made it my mission to recreate them upon returning home. I tried them as "truffles" instead of muffins (although you can press the dough into muffin liners instead). I love how the carrot shines through, and together with the dates, there is a natural sweetness (and color!) anyone will love.

ingredients

- 1 cup raw walnuts or pecans
- 12–14 Medjool dates, pitted
  (equals about 1 cup)
- 2 tablespoons melted coconut oil
- 1½ cup shredded carrots
  (about 2 large carrots)
- 1 teaspoon cinnamon
- ½ teaspoon freshly grated ginger or
  ginger powder
- ½ teaspoon nutmeg

directions

1. Place the raw walnuts or pecans in a food processor. Blend until the consistency of coarse sand. Add the dates and coconut oil, and process again until a sticky dough is formed.

2. Add the shredded carrots to the food processor and blend again until they are incorporated into the dough. Add the cinnamon, ginger, and nutmeg, and process again until all ingredients are blended.

3. Using a 1½-inch cookie scoop or your hands, roll the dough into balls of desired size (about 1 to 2 inches in diameter). Repeat until all of the dough is used up, placing them on a plate or cutting board, or in a shallow dish. Transfer them to the refrigerator to chill, at least 2 hours. You can also place them in the freezer for 30 minutes.

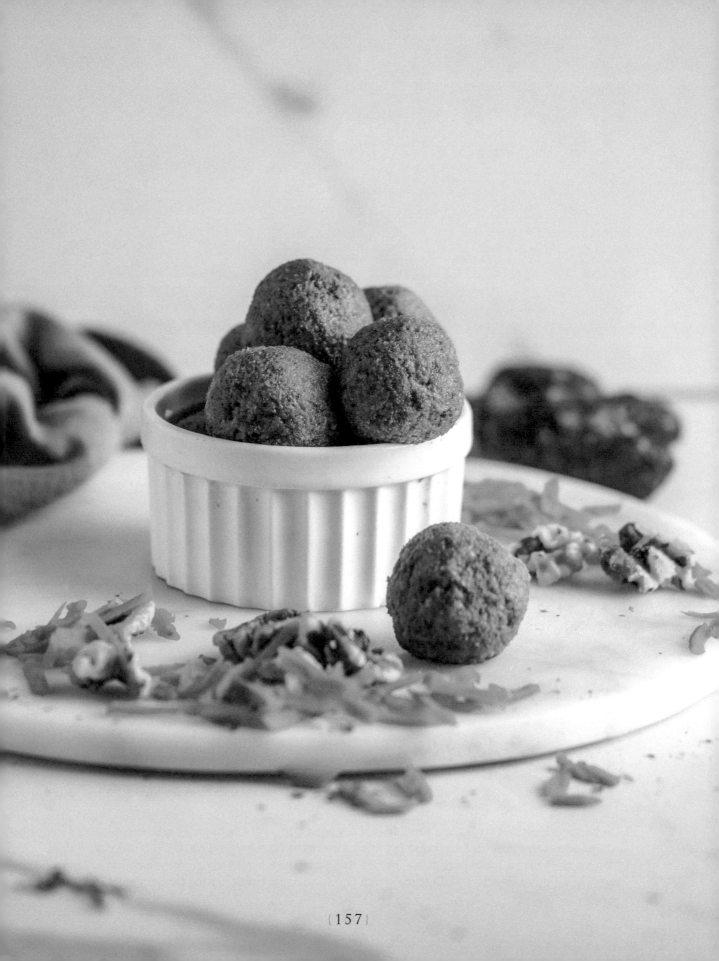

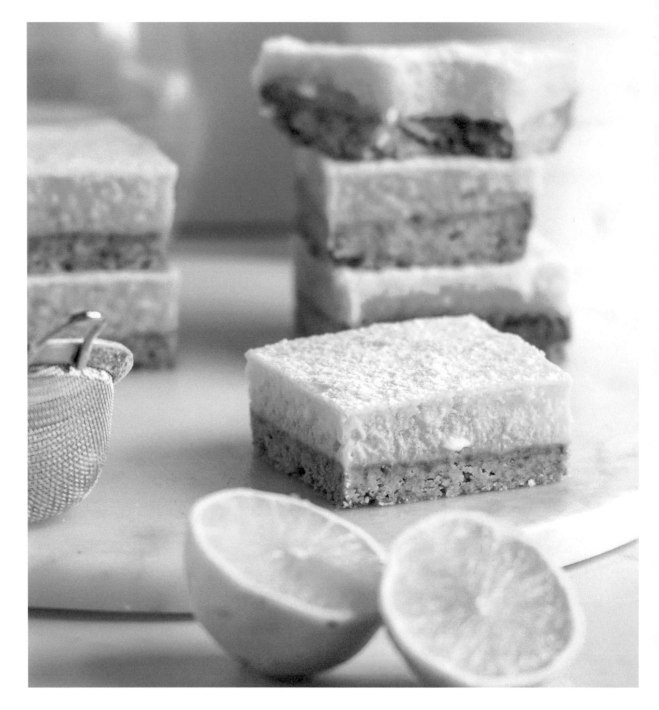

lemon squares

Makes 9 servings

I will be honest, when it comes to a sweet treat, I am not a citrus person, but my key lime pie-loving husband adores this dessert. I wanted to put this recipe in the book because when you think of a lemon square, you can't help but smile—they are so sunny! The vibrant yellow color will definitely have you eating with your eyes as well. Dust them with powdered sugar before serving for extra presentation.

ingredients

FOR THE CRUST:

- 1½ cup almond flour
- ¼ cup coconut sugar (or granulated sugar of choice)
- ¼ cup tapioca flour or arrowroot starch
- ½ cup melted coconut oil, vegan butter, or grass-fed butter
- 1 teaspoon vanilla extract

FOR THE LEMON FILLING:

- 4 large eggs
- 1½ cup white granulated sugar (see note)
- 1 tablespoon lemon zest (about 2 lemons)
- 1 cup lemon juice (about 6 medium lemons)
- 2 tablespoons arrowroot starch
- Powdered monk fruit or sugar for dusting (optional)

directions

1. Preheat the oven to 350° F. Line an 8" x 8" baking pan with parchment paper.

2. Make the crust: In a medium mixing bowl, combine the almond flour, granulated sugar, and starch. Stir to blend. In a separate small bowl, whisk together the melted oil or butter and vanilla extract. Pour the wet mixture into the bowl with the dry ingredients. Use a spatula or wooden spoon to stir until a dough is formed (it should feel like the consistency of damp sand). Use your hands to press the dough evenly into the bottom of the baking pan. Pre-bake the crust for 20 to 25 minutes, until it is slightly firmer to the touch and starting to turn golden brown. Set aside until ready to use. Decrease the oven temperature to 325° F.

3. While the crust is baking, prepare the lemon filling. In a medium pot, whisk together the eggs, granulated sugar, and lemon zest. Whisk in lemon juice, and heat everything over low heat, stirring constantly (but not vigorously) for about 3 to 5 minutes. Increase the heat to medium, and continue to stir until the mixture is hot, about 6 to 8 minutes. Turn off the heat, and add the arrowroot starch, whisking vigorously until blended and the mixture has started to thicken, about 30 seconds. There might still be some small clumps, but that is OK.

4. Transfer the egg and lemon mixture to the baking dish over the pre-baked crust. Cover with aluminum foil and bake for 10 to 12 minutes. Take the baking dish from the oven, remove the foil, and allow to completely cool at room temperature for 2 hours. Transfer to the refrigerator to further set, about 1 to 2 more hours.

5. When ready to serve, dust with powdered sugar if desired and slice into squares. Serve chilled.

notes

» *When I first tested this recipe, I used coconut sugar in the filling, and while I could tell it was sweet enough, it turned the mixture brown. I wanted to maintain the yellow hue, so if you feel the same, only a white granulated sugar will do. For the most blood sugar balancing options, use allulose or erythritol; otherwise, use regular white sugar.*

» *Remember to zest your lemons before juicing.*

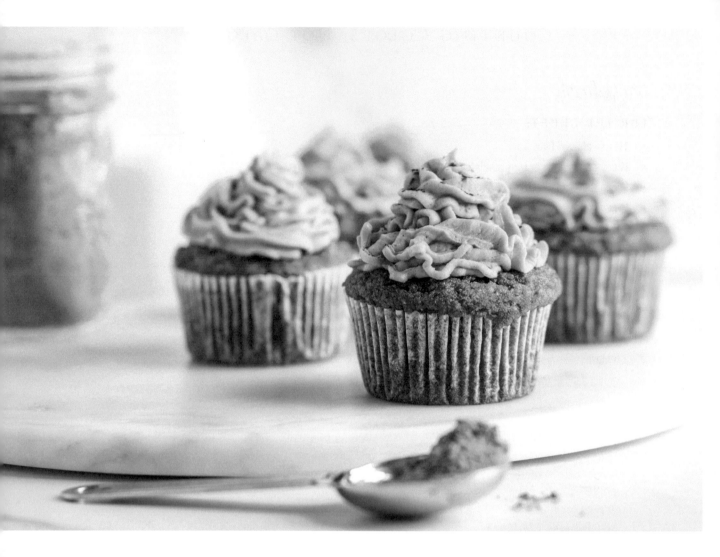

vanilla cupcakes
WITH MATCHA FROSTING

Makes 10 to 12 servings

The frosting is my favorite part of a cupcake, and the green hue highlights it here in this recipe. Sometimes it only takes one nutrient-dense ingredient to make a dish or dessert colorful. Matcha, a powdered green tea, is popular in the wellness world. It contains a class of polyphenolic compounds called catechins, an antioxidant known for its anti-inflammatory and disease-fighting properties. A tablespoon is all you need in this recipe to add the benefits to this delicious sweet treat.

ingredients

FOR THE CUPCAKES:

- 2 cups almond flour
- ¾ cup coconut sugar
- ¼ cup coconut flour

- ¼ cup tapioca flour
- 1 teaspoon baking powder
- ½ teaspoon baking soda
- ¼ teaspoon sea salt
- ½ cup dairy-free milk of choice
- 2 eggs beaten
- ½ cup unsweetened applesauce
- ¼ cup maple syrup
- 1 teaspoon vanilla extract

FOR THE FROSTING:

- ½ cup coconut oil, room temperature
- ½ cup palm oil shortening, grass-fed butter, or vegan butter, room temperature
- 1 cup monk fruit powdered sugar (or substitute with regular powdered sugar)
- 1 tablespoon matcha powder
- 2 teaspoons vanilla extract

directions

1. Preheat the oven to 350° F. Line a muffin tin with cupcake liners.

2. In a large bowl or stand mixer, mix the almond flour, coconut sugar, coconut flour, tapioca flour, baking powder, baking soda, and salt. Stir to blend.

4. In a separate medium mixing bowl, whisk together the dairy-free milk, eggs, unsweetened applesauce, maple syrup, and vanilla extract until creamy.

5. Pour the wet ingredients into the bowl with the flour mixture. Beat until a batter is formed, increasing the speed as needed.

6. Transfer the batter into the cupcake liners, filling the cups about two-thirds to three-quarters full. Bake for 22 to 25 minutes, until the tops are golden brown and a toothpick inserted into the center of one comes out clean. Allow the cupcakes to slightly cool for 5 to 10 minutes in the muffin tin, before transferring them to a wire rack to cool completely before frosting, about 1 to 2 hours.

7. Make the frosting: In a large bowl, combine the coconut oil and palm oil shortening or butter. Beat with a hand mixer until fluffy, about 1 minute. You can also use a large whisk to beat by hand.

8. Add the remaining ingredients and beat again, using a spatula to scrape down the sides as needed.

9. Using a spatula, mix the frosting. Frost the cooled cupcakes immediately, or transfer the frosting to the refrigerator for 10 minutes for a denser texture.

note

» Another way to get a green frosting is to use spirulina. Instead of 1 tablespoon of matcha powder, use 1 teaspoon of spirulina.

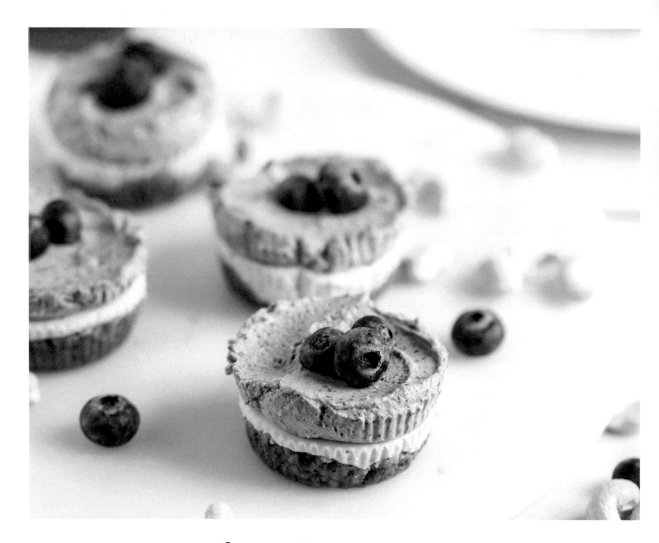

mini raw blueberry
CHEESECAKES

Makes 12 to 14 servings

While this recipe might take a bit of planning and preparing, the end result is a delightfully delicious and perfectly portioned dessert. These mini raw blueberry cheesecakes are creamy with just the right amount of sweetness. They are great to serve at a luncheon or shower, or make them for yourself when you want to satisfy your sweet tooth in a healthier way. Given that they are made with a lot of healthy fat, you will feel satisfied after eating just one. I recommend making this recipe a day or two before you plan to enjoy them, in order to give them enough time to set.

ingredients

FOR THE CRUST:

- 1½ cup raw walnuts

- 12–14 Medjool dates, pits removed

- 3 tablespoons melted coconut oil

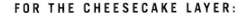

FOR THE CHEESECAKE LAYER:

- 2 cups raw cashews, soaked for at least 4–6 hours or overnight, drained and rinsed
- ¾ cup almond milk
- ⅓ cup maple syrup
- ¼ cup melted coconut oil
- 1 teaspoon vanilla extract

FOR THE BLUEBERRY LAYER:

- 1 cup raw cashews, soaked for at least 4–6 hours or overnight, drained and rinsed
- ⅓ cup almond milk
- 3 tablespoons maple syrup
- 2 tablespoons coconut oil
- 1 teaspoon vanilla extract
- 1 cup fresh blueberries

directions

1. Make the crust: Place walnuts in a food processor and blend until the consistency of coarse sand. Add the dates, and while blending, slowly incorporate the melted coconut oil until a sticky dough is formed. Using a cookie scoop, a large spoon, or your hands, press 1½ to 2 tablespoons of the dough into the bottom of muffin liners or a silicone muffin mold. Repeat until all of the dough is used, and then transfer them to the refrigerator to set.

2. Make the cheesecake layer. In a high-speed blender, combine the cashews, almond milk, maple syrup, melted coconut oil, and vanilla extract. Start blending on low, and then gradually increase to high, using the tamper to get everything in the blender going and until the mixture becomes thick and creamy.

3. Remove the muffin cups with the crust from the refrigerator. Using a cookie scoop or a large spoon, transfer 1½ to 2 tablespoons of the cashew cheesecake mixture into the individual muffin cups with the crust, making sure there is still room for the third layer (about ½ inch). Repeat until all of the muffin cups have been filled. Allow this layer to set for at least 30 minutes in the freezer or, ideally, in the refrigerator for 6–8 hours (or overnight). If you have any of the cashew cheesecake mixture left over, you can place it in an airtight container or mason jar and keep it in the refrigerator for another use (see note).

4. When the cheesecake layer has mostly set, make the blueberry layer. In a high-speed blender, combine the cashews, almond milk, maple syrup, coconut oil, vanilla extract, and blueberries. Start blending on low, and then gradually increase to high, using the tamper to get everything in the blender going.

5. Divide the blueberry mixture evenly between the muffin cups with the crust and cashew cheesecake layer. Transfer the raw cheesecakes to the freezer to set, at least 2 hours, or you can place them in the refrigerator for 4 to 6 hours (or ideally overnight). If frozen, allow the cheesecakes to sit out at room temperature for 15 to 20 minutes to slightly thaw before serving.

note

» Any leftover middle cheesecake layer is "cashew cream." It makes a delicious plant-based yogurt or topping. Enjoy with granola or spoon it over your breakfast bowl.

avocado cacao mousse

Makes 4 servings

I debated whether to include this recipe in this book, mostly because the base of this dessert isn't very colorful at all. But I am a chocolate lover through and through, and to have a dessert section with no chocolate would be sad to me. While the end result turns out to be brown, you know you are using a green ingredient (avocado), so there's that. Plus, the addition raspberries and crushed pistachios on top does add a punch of color. If you love chocolate as much as I do, you will love this silky avocado cacao mousse.

ingredients

- 3 ripe large avocados
- ½ cup raw cacao powder or cocoa powder
- ¼ cup coconut cream
- ¼ cup maple syrup
- 1 teaspoon vanilla extract
- 2 tablespoons crushed pistachios (optional)
- 1 cup fresh raspberries (optional)

directions

1. In a high-speed blender or food processor, combine the avocado, raw cacao or cocoa powder, coconut cream, maple syrup, and vanilla extract. Start blending on medium, gradually increasing the speed to high. (If you are using a Vitamix, use the tamper to get everything going.) Use a spatula to scrape down the sides, and blend until the consistency is smooth and creamy.

2. Transfer the mousse to an airtight container, and allow it to chill in the refrigerator for at least an hour. It tastes even better the next day after chilling in the refrigerator overnight!

3. To serve, top with crushed pistachios and raspberries if desired.

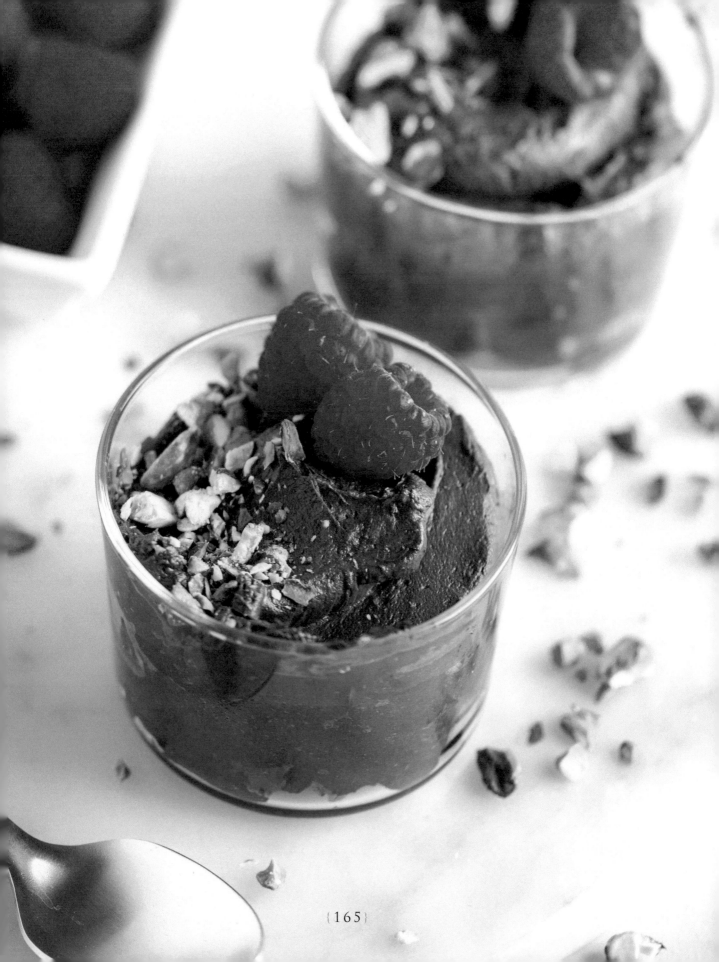

acknowledgements

Publishing *Counting Colors* wouldn't have been possible without the following, for whom I am so grateful.

To my health coaching clients, it all started with you. In our work together, you taught me so much about what it means to be healthy and happy. How wellness runs deeper than exercise, nutrition, and a number you see on a scale. Your journeys demonstrated the power of commitment, self-love, and alignment, and is the true inspiration behind this book. Thank you for trusting me in the process.

Kate Stephenson, your help with the recipes got me over a very big block I had around this book's process. I don't think I would have finished it without you. Your creativity and talent in both recipe creating and cooking, coupled with your commitment to nutritious, colorful food is inspiring. I am lucky to call you a colleague and a friend, and it was an honor to work with you.

Brandy and Matt Shay, thank you for helping to make my Counting Colors dream come true. Brandy, I am so thankful our paths crossed with my first cookbook - I remember telling you about the "Counting Colors" concept on our very first call, and six years later here we are. Thank you for believing in me and this project.

Ellie Burke, you are so much more than my life coach – you are my friend, mentor, and someone I look up to most. While I don't know if I would have accomplished half of what I wanted to without your guidance, most importantly, you helped me believe in myself, which is the greatest gift. Thank you for all of your support over the years.

Most importantly, to my family, Alex and Mason. If it wasn't for your love and support, I would have given up on this dream project a long time ago. Alex, thank you for encouraging me to not only start, but also to keep going; for reading, editing, and cheering me on along the way. Your commitment to your own creativity has been a true inspiration to this process. Mason, becoming your mom drove a deeper motivational "why" behind everything that I do. I love you.

REFERENCES

Introduction

[1] Roth, Geneen. (2011). *Women, Food, and God.* New York, NY: Scribner.

[2] Brown, Brene. (2018). *Dare to Lead: Brave Work. Tough Conversations. Whole Hearts.* New York, NY: Random House Publishing Group.

[3] (2007). *A Course in Miracles: Combined Volume.* 3rd ed. Mill Valley, CA: Foundation for Inner Peace.

Chapter One: The Influence of Story

[4] Johnson, Susan M. (2008). *Hold Me Tight: Seven Conversations for a Lifetime of Love.* New York, NY: Little, Brown & Co.

[5] Mohr, Tara. (2014). *Playing Big: Practical Wisdom for Women Who Want to Speak Up, Create, and Lead.* New York, NY: Penguin Publishing Group.

[6] Quittkat, H. L., Hartmann, A. S., Düsing, R., Buhlmann, U., & Vocks, S. (2019). Body Dissatisfaction, Importance of Appearance, and Body Appreciation in Men and Women Over the Lifespan. *Frontiers in Psychiatry*, 10(864). https://doi.org/10.3389/fpsyt.2019.00864

[7] Roth, Geneen. (2011). *Women, Food, and God.* New York, NY: Scribner.

[8] Sarno, John E. (1998). *The Mindbody Prescription: Healing the Body, Healing the Pain.* New York, NY: Grand Central Publishing.

Chapter Two: A New Model of Thinking and Believing

[9] Castillo, Brooke. (Host). (2014, October 9). The Self-Coaching Model (No. 26) [Audio Podcast episode]. In *The Life Coach School.* https://thelifecoachschool.com/podcast/26/

[10] Bernstein, G. (2019). *Super Attractor: Methods for Manifesting a Life beyond Your Wildest Dreams.* New York, NY: Hay House Inc.

[11] Achor, S. (2012). Positive Intelligence. Three ways individuals can cultivate their own sense of well-being and set themselves up to succeed. *Harvard Business Review, Vol. 90, Issue ½.* https://www.dea.univr.it/documenti/OccorrenzaIns/matdid/matdid467193.pdf.

Chapter Three: Upshifting to Neutrality with Nutritional Science

[12] Jensen, J., Rustad, P. I., Kolnes, A. J., & Lai, Y.-C. (2011). The Role of Skeletal Muscle Glycogen Breakdown for Regulation of Insulin Sensitivity by Exercise. *Frontiers in Physiology*, 2(112). https://doi.org/10.3389/fphys.2011.00112

[13] Lan, Y.-L., Lou, J.-C., Lyu, W., & Zhang, B. (2019). Update on the synergistic effect of HSL and insulin in the treatment of metabolic disorders. *Therapeutic Advances in Endocrinology and Metabolism*, 10, 204201881987730. https://doi.org/10.1177/2042018819877300

[14] Amin, T., & Mercer, J. G. (2016). Hunger and Satiety Mechanisms and Their Potential Exploitation in the Regulation of Food Intake. *Current Obesity Reports*, 5(1), 106–112. https://doi.org/10.1007/s13679-015-0184-5

[15] Lim, S. (n.d.). *Research suggests stress only damages your health if you think it does.* Business Insider. https://www.businessinsider.com/research-suggests-stress-only-damages-your-health-if-you-think-it-does-2018-9

[16] Keller, A., Litzelman, K., Wisk, L. E., Maddox, T., Cheng, E. R., Creswell, P. D., & Witt, W. P. (2012). Does the perception that stress affects health matter? The association with health and mortality. *Health Psychology*, 31(5), 677–684. https://doi.org/10.1037/a0026743

[17] Mcgonigal, K. (2016). *The Upside of Stress: Why Stress Is Good for You, and How to Get Good at It.* New York, NY: Avery.

[18] Kuo, T., McQueen, A., Chen, T.-C., & Wang, J.-C. (2015). Regulation of Glucose Homeostasis by Glucocorticoids. *Advances in Experimental Medicine and Biology*, 872, 99–126. https://doi.org/10.1007/978-1-4939-2895-8_5

[19] Barclay, G. R., & Turnberg, L. A. (1987). Effect of psychological stress on salt and water transport in the human jejunum. *Gastroenterology*, 93(1), 91–97. https://doi.org/10.1016/0016-5085(87)90319-2

[20] David, M. (2015). *The Slow Down Diet: Eating for Pleasure, Energy, and Weight*. Rochester, VT: Healing Arts Press.

[21] Konturek PC, Brzozowski T, Konturek SJ. Stress and the gut: pathophysiology, clinical consequences, diagnostic approach and treatment options. J Physiol Pharmacol. 2011 Dec;62(6):591-9. PMID: 22314561. https://pubmed.ncbi.nlm.nih.gov/22314561/

[22] Dispenza, J. (2019). *Becoming Supernatural: How Common People are Doing the Uncommon*. New York, NY: Hay House Inc.

Chapter Four: Meals as a Microcosm of Mindfulness

[23] Barclay, G. R., & Turnberg, L. A. (1987). *Effect of psychological stress on salt and water transport in the human jejunum. Gastroenterology*, 93(1), 91–97. https://doi.org/10.1016/0016-5085(87)90319-2

[24] Baldaro, B., Battacchi, M. W., Trombini, G., Palomba, D., & Stegagno, L. (1990). Effects of an Emotional Negative Stimulus on the Cardiac, Electrogastrographic, and Respiratory Responses. *Perceptual and Motor Skills*, 71(2), 647–655. https://doi.org/10.2466/pms.1990.71.2.647

[25] (2007). *A Course in Miracles: Combined Volume*. 3rd ed. Mill Valley, CA: Foundation for Inner Peace.

[26] Brady, L. S., Smith, M. A., Gold, P. W., & Herkenham, M. (1990). Altered Expression of Hypothalamic Neuropeptide mRNAs in Food-Restricted and Food-Deprived Rats. *Neuroendocrinology*, 52(5), 441–447. https://doi.org/10.1159/000125626

[27] Beck, B. (2006). Neuropeptide Y in normal eating and in genetic and dietary-induced obesity. *Philosophical Transactions of the Royal Society B: Biological Sciences*, 361(1471), 1159–1185. https://doi.org/10.1098/rstb.2006.1855

[28] Kabat-Zinn, J., & Amazon.com (Firm. (2009). *Wherever You Go, There You Are: Mindfulness Meditation in Everyday Life*. New York, NY: Hachette Books.

Chapter Five: The Power of Your Thoughts

[29] Singer, M. A. (2007). *The Untethered Soul: The Journey Beyond Yourself*. Oakland, CA: New Harbinger Publications, Inc.

[30] Clapp, M., Aurora, N., Herrera, L., Bhatia, M., Wilen, E., & Wakefield, S. (2017). Gut microbiota's effect on mental health: the gut-brain axis. *Clinics and Practice*, 7(4). https://doi.org/10.4081/cp.2017.987

Chapter Six: Practicing the Art of Non-Judgment

[31] Sarno, John E. (1998). *The Mindbody Prescription: Healing the Body, Healing the Pain*. New York, NY: Grand Central Publishing.

[32] Loewenstein, G. (1994). The psychology of curiosity: A review and reinterpretation. *Psychological Bulletin*, 116(1), 75–98. https://doi.org/10.1037/0033-2909.116.1.75

[33] Schott, B. H., Minuzzi, L., Krebs, R. M., Elmenhorst, D., Lang, M., Winz, O. H., Seidenbecher, C. I., Coenen, H. H., Heinze, H.-J. ., Zilles, K., Duzel, E., & Bauer, A. (2008). Mesolimbic Functional Magnetic Resonance Imaging Activations during Reward Anticipation Correlate with Reward-Related Ventral Striatal Dopamine Release. *Journal of Neuroscience*, 28(52), 14311–14319. https://doi.org/10.1523/jneurosci.2058-08.2008

34 Williamson, M. (1996). *A Return to Love: Reflections on the Principles of a Course in Miracles*. New York, NY: HarperOne.

35 Kubler-Ross, E. & Kessler, D. (2001). *Life Lessons: Two Experts on Death and Dying Teach Us About the Mysteries of Life and Living*. New York, NY: Scribner.

36 David, M. (2015). *The Slow Down Diet: Eating for Pleasure, Energy, and Weight*. Rochester, VT: Healing Arts Press.

37 Lipton, B. H. (2016). *The Biology of Belief: Unleashing the Power of Consciousness, Matter and Miracles*. New York, NY: Hay House, Inc.

38 Roth, Geneen. (2011). *Women, Food, and God*. New York, NY: Scribner.

39 Dispenza, J. (2015). *You Are the Placebo: Making Your Mind Matter*. New York, NY: Hay House, Inc.

40 National Science Foundation. (2005). NSF - *National Science Foundation*. https://www.nsf.gov/

41 Kolb, B., Gibb, R., & Robinson, T. E. (2003). Brain Plasticity and Behavior. *Current Directions in Psychological Science*, 12(1), 1–5. https://doi.org/10.1111/1467-8721.01210

Chapter Seven: Rewrite Your Health Story

42 Singer, M. A. (2007). *The Untethered Soul: The Journey Beyond Yourself*. Oakland, CA: New Harbinger Publications, Inc.

43 Stutz, P. & Michels, B. *The Tools: 5 Tools to Help You Find Courage, Creativity, and Willpower—and Inspire You to Live Life in Forward Motion*. New York, NY: Random House.

44 Clear, J. (2018). *Atomic Habits*. New York, NY: Penguin Publishing Group.

45 Kabat-Zinn, J., & Amazon.com (Firm. (2009). *Wherever You Go, There You Are: Mindfulness Meditation in Everyday Life*. New York, NY: Hachette Books.

46 Katie, B., & Mitchell, S. (2003). *Loving What Is: Four Questions That Can Change Your Life*. New York, NY: Harmony/Rodale.

47 Hendricks, G. (2010). *The Big Leap: Conquer Your Hidden Fear and Take Life to the Next Level*. New York, NY: HarperCollins.

Chapter Eight: The Law of Attraction and Manifestation

48 Canfield, J. (2007). *The Success Principles*. New York, NY: HarperCollins.

49 Jung, M., & Lee, M. (2021). The Effect of a Mindfulness-Based Education Program on Brain Waves and the Autonomic Nervous System in University Students. *Healthcare, 9*(11), 1606. https://doi.org/10.3390/healthcare9111606

50 Castillo, B. & Stevenson, C. (2011). *It Was Always Meant to Happen That Way*. Futures Unlimited.

51 Li, J.-J., Dou, K., Wang, Y.-J., & Nie, Y.-G. (2019). Why Awe Promotes Prosocial Behaviors? The Mediating Effects of Future Time Perspective and Self-Transcendence Meaning of Life. *Frontiers in Psychology, 10*. https://doi.org/10.3389/fpsyg.2019.01140

52 Jiang, T., & Sedikides, C. (2021). Awe motivates authentic-self pursuit via self-transcendence: Implications for prosociality. *Journal of Personality and Social Psychology*. https://doi.org/10.1037/pspi0000381

53 Hendricks, G. (2021). *The Genius Zone: The Breakthrough Process to End Negative Thinking and Live in True Creativity*. New York, NY: St. Martin's Press.

Chapter Nine: The Power of Belief

54 Kaptchuk, T. J., Friedlander, E., Kelley, J. M., Sanchez, M. N., Kokkotou, E., Singer, J. P., Kowalczykowski, M., Miller, F. G., Kirsch, I., & Lembo, A. J. (2010). Placebos without Deception: A Randomized Controlled Trial in Irritable Bowel Syndrome. *PLoS ONE, 5*(12), e15591. https://doi.org/10.1371/journal.pone.0015591

[55] Baylor College Of Medicine. (2002, July 12). Study Finds Common Knee Surgery No Better Than Placebo. *ScienceDaily*. Retrieved October 4, 2022 from www.sciencedaily.com/releases/2002/07/020712075415.htm

[56] Crum, A. J., & Langer, E. J. (2007). Mind-Set Matters. *Psychological Science*, 18(2), 165–171. https://doi.org/10.1111/j.1467-9280.2007.01867.x

[57] Tolle, E. (2004). The Power of Now: *A Guide to Spiritual Enlightenment*. Novato, CA: Namaste Publishing.

[58] Canfield, J. (2007). *The Success Principles*. New York, NY: HarperCollins.

Chapter Ten: Create Your Own Reality and Find Your Flow

[59] Tachon, G., Shankland, R., Marteau-Chasserieau, F., Morgan, B., Leys, C., & Kotsou, I. (2021). Gratitude Moderates the Relation between Daily Hassles and Satisfaction with Life in University Students. *International Journal of Environmental Research and Public Health*, 18(24), 13005. https://doi.org/10.3390/ijerph182413005

[60] Wood, A. M., Froh, J. J., & Geraghty, A. W. A. (2010). Gratitude and well-being: A review and theoretical integration. *Clinical Psychology Review*, 30(7), 890–905. https://doi.org/10.1016/j.cpr.2010.03.005

[61] Wilson, T. D., Reinhard, D. A., Westgate, E. C., Gilbert, D. T., Ellerbeck, N., Hahn, C., Brown, C. L., & Shaked, A. (2014). Just think: The challenges of the disengaged mind. *Science*, 345(6192), 75–77. https://doi.org/10.1126/science.1250830

[62] Fisher, H. E., Brown, L. L., Aron, A., Strong, G., & Mashek, D. (2010). Reward, Addiction, and Emotion Regulation Systems Associated With Rejection in Love. *Journal of Neurophysiology*, 104(1), 51–60. https://doi.org/10.1152/jn.00784.2009

[63] Pomrenze, M. B., Giovanetti, S. M., Maiya, R., Gordon, A. G., Kreeger, L. J., & Messing, R. O. (2019). Dissecting the Roles of GABA and Neuropeptides from Rat Central Amygdala CRF Neurons in Anxiety and Fear Learning. *Cell Reports*, 29(1), 13-21.e4. https://doi.org/10.1016/j.celrep.2019.08.083

[64] Comeras, L. B., Herzog, H., & Tasan, R. O. (2019). Neuropeptides at the crossroad of fear and hunger: a special focus on neuropeptide Y. *Annals of the New York Academy of Sciences*, 1455(1), 59–80. https://doi.org/10.1111/nyas.14179

[65] McNamara, M. E. (2022). Neuroplasticity, change and addiction disorders. *Neurological Science Journal*. 6:1.

[66] Dispenza, J., & Amen, D. G. (2015). *Breaking the Habit of Being Yourself: How to Lose Your Mind and Create a New One*. New York, NY: Hay House.

[67] Killingsworth, M. A., & Gilbert, D. T. (2010). A Wandering Mind Is an Unhappy Mind. *Science*, 330(6006), 932–932. https://doi.org/10.1126/science.1192439

[68] Cruikshank, T. (2016). *Meditate Your Weight: A 21-Day Retreat to Optimize Your Metabolism and Feel Great*. New York, NY: Harmony.

[69] Egbert, M. D., & Barandiaran, X. E. (2014). Modeling habits as self-sustaining patterns of sensorimotor behavior. *Frontiers in Human Neuroscience*, 8. https://doi.org/10.3389/fnhum.2014.00590

[70] Williamson, M. (1996). *A Return to Love: Reflections on the Principles of a Course in Miracles*. New York, NY: HarperOne.

Made in United States
Troutdale, OR
11/24/2024

25269738R00102